MW01241958

Dr Joannou has written a v
tion to guide the reader to a
is, how it is diagnosed and options for treatment. The book is very clearly
set out and the 'How to Use this Book' chapter is a gem. It allows the reader
to go straight to the answers for whatever burning questions they may have.
Along the way the author also explores some very important issues such as
the inappropriate medicalisation of certain aspects of normal human experience such as grief and anxiety. Every chapter is meticulously supported by
references, providing the reader with further resources to pursue. Above all,
what shines through the pages of this book is the compassion and humanity
of the author who clearly cares deeply for the wellbeing of his patients, and
who extends this to his readers. I heartily recommend this book to anybody
who wants to have a deeper understanding of depression, whether it be for
themselves or someone they care about.

Dr John McDonald, PhD
(Registered acupuncturist, author, academic and researcher)

I have personally observed Dr Alex in his clinical studies with Anxiety and
Depression and witnessed phenomenal results. His clinical expertise as
a long-standing GP in combination with acupuncture, a tried and tested
healing modality, is a powerful union. I highly recommend this informative
book which will give the reader hope that there are natural alternatives, or as
an adjunct to conventional medicine for those with mental health problems.

Adam O'Mara BHS-Acu, Acupuncturist 13 years

In his second publication on depression, Dr Alex Joannou presents a
well-organised, well argued and knowledgeable publication in support of
his powerful message: Transformational Acupuncture benefits depression
sufferers. Beneficial to both doctors and clients, Dr Joannou provides
numerous case studies in support of his argument. This book is well worth
the read.

Dr J. A. Swain, BA(Hons) PhD

Dr. Alexander Joannou is courageously paving the way for the future of medicine and the treatment of depression. In fact, I'd dare say, the future is now. Acupuncture is both natural and effective for helping people to activate their body's natural ability to heal. I highly recommend *Stick it to Depression*, because I know it works.

Dr. Darren Weissman,
Best selling author of *Awakening to the Secret Code of Your Mind* and Developer of The LifeLine Technique®

A truly beautiful book about the art of healing! Dr Alexander Joannou suffered a chronic life threatening disease that opened his world to different healing methods to consider and address deeper causes for his illness. This personal journey made him a better, more compassionate doctor to help serve his patients. He now so generously shares his skills and knowledge with case studies of his own patients. I was particularly inspired by his wisdom of the various healing disciplines available whether they are acupuncture, nutritional medicine or mind-body medicine to help heal the patient as a whole: "... the various traditions and techniques allow us to see human beings from a different perspective. Each discipline has its own language to describe what is going on within us. Each discipline has its own strengths and its own weaknesses. None of these disciplines, including conventional Western medicine, can describe the totality of what is going on within each one of us."

Associate Professor Vicki Kotsirilos AM,
MBBS, Awarded Honorary Fellow of the RACGP, FACNEM, FASLM
Holistic GP, Academic, Media commentator, Researcher, Writer

STICK IT TO
DEPRESSION

Get your life back, *naturally*

DR ALEXANDER JOANNOU

First published 2021 by Alexander Joannou

Produced by Indie Experts P/L, Australasia
indieexperts.com.au

Cover design by Daniela Catucci @ Catucci Design
Edited by Lauren Mitchell
Internal design by Indie Experts
Typeset in 11.5/15 pt Adobe Garamond Pro by Post Pre-press Group, Brisbane

A catalogue record for this book is available from the National Library of Australia

ISBN 978-0-6487018-3-5 (paperback)
ISBN 978-0-6487018-4-2 (epub)
ISBN 978-0-6487018-5-9 (kindle)

Disclaimer:
The content of this book is for informational purposes only and is not intended to diagnose, treat, cure, or prevent any condition or disease. You understand that this book is not intended as a substitute for consultation with a licensed practitioner. Please consult with your own physician or healthcare specialist regarding the suggestions and recommendations made in this book. The use of this book implies your acceptance of this disclaimer.

For Mikio,
the giant on whose shoulders I have stood

CONTENTS

IF YOU OR SOMEONE YOU KNOW IS IN CRISIS PLEASE CALL
ONE OF THE FOLLOWING AUSTRALIAN NATIONAL HELPLINES:
LIFELINE AUSTRALIA – 13 11 14
SUICIDE CALL BACK SERVICE – 1300 659 467

PREFACE

THE PROBLEM OF DEPRESSION

'I felt a total lack of joy in my life. I would just go and lie down. Sometimes I would feel like I wanted to cry for no reason whatsoever. I think that was the last straw. That's why I came to you, because of the feelings of wanting to cry for no apparent reason. I felt a total loss of confidence.'

Eric (not his real name, which is true for all case studies I refer to in this book) was a very successful high management professional in the prime of his life. To all appearances, even to his friends, he seemed very successful in his work and a great family man. He seemed quite happy and knew what he wanted in life.

Eric said, 'In retrospect, I realise I've been depressed for about the last year and a half. It was a gradual awareness that I came to know, and finally admit to myself, that I felt like a failure. I felt shame. I felt defeated. I came to you because I knew I could get trusted medical advice. I needed to find a reason, an underlying reason, why I was depressed. I told three friends about my feeling depressed, but none of them were any help. No one tried to contact me or to catch up with me or lend a sympathetic ear.'

Jill, a mature aged widow who attained a PhD late in life, said, 'I didn't think of myself as being depressed back then. I was surrounded by people with depression, my husband, my sister, my mother – and there was bipolar in the family. I didn't feel like I was *that* bad. Not like them. But I remember thinking, is this all there is to life? Does this go on forever? I've got to get out of this. Then I remembered how I felt when I previously had acupuncture with you [for shingles pain], so I booked in to see you.'

A third patient, Kate, said, 'I've been depressed most of my life. With six children and a grumpy husband, I relied on Valium to get me through the day. I didn't want to do anything. I pushed myself to get out of bed each day.'

A fourth patient, Ray: 'The central question for me was how to not become a victim of my own depression. It was just too easy to blame the depression and just keep staying where I was.'

And a final patient, Chewie, another great family man whom I have known for a long time, felt totally defeated: 'I felt like I was evaporating away. There'd been a lot of problems at home with a teenager. When my car broke down, it felt like it was the straw that broke the camel's back. I felt like in some way I'd wronged God. I felt broken. I wasn't able to sleep. I wasn't able to focus. I felt strange inside. I thought I was having a heart attack. I booked an appointment to see my minister, but he forgot to turn up. How bad is that? I felt so unworthy. I couldn't fight anymore. I felt catatonic. My wife and children were pleading with me. They loved me and needed me and said that I was worth something to them. But I didn't listen. Couldn't listen. I didn't know where I went wrong. I felt angry and frustrated – with myself, with God. I didn't care if I died. When members of my family were killed in a horrific car smash years ago, that time was bad. The inquest was awful. But you know what? This depression was worse. I never felt as hopeless in my whole life.'

If you can relate to *these* stories, or you have close friends or family who can relate to these stories, then this book is for you. In this book I'll talk about the problem of depression, what it means for the world, and what it means for you as an individual. I'll describe what depression is, how it is diagnosed, and the options to treat it.

The medical profession, and the Western world in general, tend to view drugs as a solution, *the* solution for everything. Western medicine does well in so many areas, particularly in emergency and trauma medicine and surgery, but one area it does not do well in, I believe, is the treatment of depression. Drugs may help, and may even be life saving for some, but I do not see them as the sole solution for depression, especially mild to moderate depression. The one thing drugs don't generally do is help people to help themselves.

My aim in writing this book is to help you to help yourself. I will do this by helping you to understand what depression is – and what it isn't. Whether you are currently on antidepressants or not, there are strategies that work, strategies that you can implement yourself to help you get your life back on track. I will explain what these strategies are.

I strongly caution anyone on antidepressants *NOT* to stop them without medical advice and only cease medication with the express recommendation and guidance of your medical practitioner. Any withdrawal from antidepressant drugs needs to be gradual and under medical supervision. I can't emphasise this enough. With that in mind, please read on.

Transformational Acupuncture is a twenty-first century development of an ancient technique. I believe that it may help in the treatment of depression, as well as reduce anxiety and stress. I have been performing acupuncture for the past twenty years and it has become a favourite tool in my doctor's bag for helping people with mental health issues. Many of my patients have generously shared their experiences, and their stories are included as case histories (with names changed).

Now, just to give you a brief taste of what is in store, I conclude this preface with the comments of just six of my patients who have experienced a course of this treatment:

'This has been the most awesome experience. I don't know why I didn't do this ages ago.' – 51-YEAR-OLD FEMALE

'I find it a lot easier to hold space for people now.' – 32-YEAR-OLD FEMALE

'I'm not so in my head now. I've got a lot better perspective. I'm not foggy.' – 37-YEAR-OLD FEMALE

'I've had two big shifts. Firstly, I don't lose my temper anymore. I don't shout at the kids. I'm much more tolerant of them. Secondly, I feel much more loving towards my husband. I haven't told him what's been happening. I keep taking him by surprise. I don't think he's sure what's going on.' – 42-YEAR-OLD FEMALE

'Oh my goodness, this is a great feeling'! – 45-YEAR-OLD MALE AFTER HIS FIRST TREATMENT

'I'm doing all these things I haven't done for a long time; I'm reading for pleasure now as I can focus; I've restarted long distance swimming, baking and cooking and just loving life.' – 52-YEAR-OLD FEMALE AFTER SIX WEEKS

It is because of comments like these from my patients every week that I feel compelled to share my knowledge with you.

Dr Alex

HOW TO USE THIS BOOK

I wrote this book in what I think is a logical order, starting with Chapter 1 outlining how big a problem depression is. But you can go straight to any chapter depending on what you need to know right now. Here is a guide:

- If you want to know how I stumbled across acupuncture as a treatment for depression go straight to Chapter 2: Acupuncture Serendipity
- If you want to understand how doctors diagnose depression, go straight to Chapter 3: What is Depression? – The Modern Medical Approach.
- If you are wondering if you are having side effects from your medication, go straight to Chapter 4: The Solution: Pills, Pills, Pills.
- If you want to know about my background, go straight to Chapter 5: What Crohn's Disease Taught Me About the Modern Medical Model.
- If you want to understand a broader approach to ill-health, go straight to Chapter 6: Body Maps – Where East Meets West
- If you want to know how doctors measure how severe your symptoms of depression are, go straight to Chapter 7: What is a DASS?
- If you are in desperate need of hope, go straight to Chapter 8: Case Studies.
- If you want some self-help strategies go straight to Chapter 9: Changing the Psychology of Depression – What Can I Do to Help Myself?
- If you are already convinced and keen to have acupuncture, but have some specific concerns, go to Chapter 10: Acupuncture FAQs.

And if you're ready to take action, check out these resources:

- If you're sold on acupuncture, where can you go to get it?
  - Go to the Australian Medical Acupuncture College website (www.amac.org.au) and click 'Find Medical Acupuncturist'; or
  - go to the Australian Acupuncture and Chinese Medicine Association website (www.acupuncture.org.au) and click 'Find a Practitioner'.
- If you're really keen to try Transformational Acupuncture, where can you find an acupuncturist specifically trained in this method?
  - Go to the Transformational Acupuncture International website (www.tai.healthcare) and click 'Find a Licenced Transformational Acupuncturist Near Me'.

1

HUMANITY'S NUMBER-ONE HEALTH PROBLEM

IT'S OFFICIAL …

I had been practicing medicine as a family physician for 16 years when I commenced practising acupuncture in 1998. Coincidentally, that same year the World Health Organization (WHO) released the Global Burden of Disease study.[1]

The study pointed out that in 1990 there were 50 million people in the world with depression. It further predicted that by the year 2020, depression would be the second leading cause of disease burden throughout the world.

Well, it's official. On 30 March 2017, WHO announced that depression is not the *second* leading cause but *the* leading cause of ill health and disability in the whole world. That is to say, the burden in terms of financial cost and the amount of time lost to depression is greater than any other medical condition.

Depression came in three years ahead of schedule and as well it has pipped coronary heart disease for the number-one position. There are over 300 million people worldwide living with depression. That is *six* times what that number was a generation ago.

The numbers are just absolutely mind boggling – and even when you look at the Australian figures, it continues to be mind boggling. In Australia at any time, one million people live with depression and two million people live with anxiety.

It is estimated that 45 per cent of Australians will experience a mental health condition in their lifetime. So, what that means is that nearly one out of every two people you pass in the street, sit next to in the football stadium or sit next to on public transport either have had, will have or currently have a mental health condition. This seems inconceivable in the lucky country, the land of plenty.

Currently eight Australians die every day by suicide. Six out of those eight are men. This is not surprising when men find it more difficult than women to ask for help.

Only one in five men with chronic mental health issues will consult a general practitioner.[2]

I confirmed this fact having recently reviewed a list of my patients coming to me for treatment of depression and anxiety. Only 20 per cent of them are males.

I could go on with the statistics and even discuss the huge economic impact on the country in terms of the costs of treatment as well as lost productivity. But the human cost is enormous.

Depression has a direct effect on the immediate family, extended family, friends and colleagues. Paula, at 36, withdrew from her family and close friends.

'I went into hibernation mode,' Paula said. 'I felt an incredible amount of shame and guilt about feeling the way I did, but I didn't have the energy to care about what anyone else was thinking. It took me all my time to drag myself out of bed in the mornings and there wasn't enough energy left to have to cope with how other people around me might be feeling. I didn't want to upset or burden other people with how bad I was feeling so I isolated myself. And if they happened to be offended, then that was their problem, because the bottom line was, I had hardly enough caring for me.'

Even all my years' experience as a medical practitioner didn't prepare me when the partner of a close friend, seemingly out of the blue, committed suicide. He left his family and friends shocked and devastated. The impact on me was to drive me to looking for a real solution to the problem of depression. I have been tinkering with acupuncture as possible solution over the past ten years, resulting in the Transformational Acupuncture System. And, it has driven me to write this book, because I want everyone to be made aware of this treatment option.

COVID-19 PANDEMIC

I wrote the preceding words in late 2019. As I review this book for publication, the foreword seems a little dated. The COVID-19 pandemic has surely surpassed depression as the number-one health problem facing humanity – or has it?

Millions have caught the disease and hundreds of thousands lay dead. The economies of practically every nation on the planet have been hugely impacted. Surely this makes it the number-one health problem – or does it?

To reiterate, there are over 300 million people living with depression and 600 million people living with anxiety. Millions of people have caught COVID-19. Without underestimating the impact on whole nations and the number of deaths, the vast majority of these millions have mild-to-no symptoms. And these symptoms resolve typically within two weeks. Whereas the symptoms and impact of depression are ongoing. The symptoms can lead to suicide. The WHO estimates that one person suicides every 40 seconds in the world.[3]

Perhaps if we viewed a chart of the countries of the world with cumulative totals of depressed people and suicide figures updated daily, this would put the problem of depression front and centre. By 31 December, *each and every year,* the total suicides in the world would be around 800,000.

Consider the age of people affected. Suicides are the second leading cause of death in 15–29 year olds around the world. They are dead before they really have had much of a chance at life. Compare this to COVID-19, which has its impact mainly in the older age groups, especially those with general ill-health. I say this not to trivialise the impact of COVID-19 but to emphasise the impact of depression.

Then there is the impact on the economies of the world. WHO estimates that depression and anxiety cost the global economy USD 1 trillion in lost productivity *each year*.[4]

There is a strong association between becoming unemployed and becoming depressed, anxious, stressed and suicidal.[5] [6]

So, if anything, the impact of the pandemic will worsen the mental health of people around the world and cement depression as the leading cause of ill-health and disability globally.

ADDITIONAL DEPRESSING DATA

Depression is associated with a number of medical conditions, including these four huge problems:

i. substance abuse
ii. chronic non-cancer pain
iii. diabetes mellitus
iv. coronary heart disease.

SUBSTANCE ABUSE

Over 500,000 Australians will experience depression and a substance use disorder at the same time, at some point in their lives.[7]

Alcohol use disorder doubles the risk of developing major depressive disorder and vice versa.[8]

People with a history of depression are more than twice as likely to smoke tobacco.[9]

It also seems that people with depression find it harder to quit smoking than those who are not depressed. Apparently, in the short term nicotine helps relieve symptoms of anxiety and depression, but the kicker is that in the long term it increases symptoms of anxiety and depression.[10]

CHRONIC NON-CANCER PAIN

Rates of depression are four times higher among people with chronic non-cancer pain compared with those without. Conversely, the presence of depression and anxiety in people with chronic non-cancer pain is strongly associated with more severe pain, greater disability and poorer health-related quality of life.[11]

So, it seems that chronic pain can cause depression, and that depression can cause chronic pain to be more severe as well as more debilitating.

Then there is another double whammy. Firstly, doctors are increasingly prescribing opioid drugs (opium-like drugs such as morphine, oxycodone and fentanyl) for chronic non-cancer pain conditions such as arthritis. Secondly, as well as the potential for being addictive, these drugs themselves can cause depression.[12]

The tragedy is that patients with chronic non-cancer pain and depression are more likely than those without depression to be prescribed opioids by their well-meaning doctor, for a longer duration and at higher morphine-equivalent doses. Patients with chronic non-cancer pain and who are depressed are more likely to misuse or abuse opioids than those with chronic non-cancer pain who are not depressed.[13]

On a more positive note, turn to Case 5 in Chapter 8: Case Studies to see an example of what acupuncture can do for chronic non-cancer pain.

DIABETES MELLITUS

According to Diabetes Australia, 'Research shows that having diabetes more than doubles the risk of developing depression.'[14]

Neave, a 28-year-old female, was diagnosed with type 1 diabetes mellitus at the age of seven. Naeve wears a small, battery-operated insulin pump 24 hours a day which delivers a surge of insulin in response to eating food. According to the Juvenile Diabetes Research Foundation, 'Depression is estimated to affect one in four people with diabetes (type 1 and type 2). Adolescents with type 1 diabetes have five times the rate of depression than adolescents that do not have T1D.'[15]

Neave also has a number of different autoimmune conditions including hypothyroidism, polycystic ovarian syndrome (PCOS), seronegative rheumatoid arthritis, alopecia totalis (complete loss of hair) and has been chronically exhausted and diagnosed by an endocrinologist with chronic fatigue syndrome/ myalgic encephalomyelitis (CFS/ME). Not surprisingly, Neave also had depression.

Over the course of sixteen weekly acupuncture treatments, Naeve showed huge improvements in her levels of depression, anxiety and stress. Nine months following the course of acupuncture, Neave reported, 'I have been really good since the treatments,' and has not felt the need to have any further acupuncture sessions.

CORONARY HEART DISEASE

Depression is a risk factor for coronary heart disease in both men[16] and in women.[17]

Further, there have been three trials run to see if treating depression with antidepressants and cognitive behaviour therapy help reduce the likelihood of heart attacks. Despite improvement in depression it *did not* improve the incidence of heart attacks. See more details about this in Chapter 6: Body Maps – Where East Meets West.

Jill, from the foreword, also has a heart condition and regularly suffers from angina (heart pain). With Transformation Acupuncture treatment, she noted that not only did her depression go away, she also had far fewer angina attacks. She was able to reduce her use of nitro spray. I don't think this is coincidental as acupuncture has been shown to help reduce the number of angina attacks in patients with coronary artery disease.[18]

So, we have now seen how big a problem depression is. What actually is depression? How is it defined? How does your doctor diagnose it? These questions will be answered in Chapter 3: What is Depression? – The Modern Medical Approach. But before looking at this I would like to discuss how I came across acupuncture as a treatment option for depression.

2

ACUPUNCTURE SERENDIPITY

I studied acupuncture back in 1998 with the then Australian Medical Acupuncture Society and completed a graduate certificate in Medical Acupuncture with Monash University in 2000. Initially, I would recommend acupuncture as a last resort for my general practice patients. Most of my early patients had chronic pain from osteoarthritis in various joints and I would perform acupuncture if they were getting side effects from their painkillers, or if they were unable to take non-steroidal anti-inflammatory drugs due to poor renal function or history of stomach ulcers. I hand-picked my patients and was cautious in recommending acupuncture at first. I found that those early patients were even more enthusiastic than I was about the acupuncture. They kept coming back, telling me of the wonderful results they were getting. Many were able to significantly reduce or even stop their painkillers. It wasn't before long that they were recommending acupuncture to their friends. The size of my acupuncture practice grew rapidly. I found myself getting more and more confident as patients kept telling me how happy they were with the results. I found that I was offering acupuncture less as a last resort to my patients and more as an adjunct to their current treatment. Eventually, I was offering acupuncture as a first resort, then offering drug therapies if the response was not good enough.

I found I was treating a wide variety of medical problems, but one condition that the acupuncture wasn't really helping was mental illness. It seemed to have a reasonable sedative or calming effect, but that effect did not last. It seemed to relax people for a couple of days or sometimes for only a few hours. But it didn't last the week, even if they came back for repeated weekly treatments.

In 2010 I attended a workshop by Dr Mikio Sankey in Melbourne. At the time I was going through turbulence in my personal life. I was drawn to the workshop because it was aimed at healing the healer. Mikio is not a medical doctor but has a double PhD in alternate healing methods and hails from California. His acupuncture method is aimed at high-level meditators and his lectures are right into theosophy and Ayurvedic language rather than the language of traditional Chinese medicine. It was a long way from the language of conventional Western medicine that I had been brought up on. And I certainly wouldn't have called myself a high-level meditator. I've merely dabbled in it from time to time.

I've always had an open mind, but when I received my first acupuncture treatment I was blown away by the imagery I experienced. I saw the countryside a hundred feet below me. It was more than visual; I could *feel* that I was flying. I could feel 6-foot angelic wings beating slowly and rhythmically. I experienced the sensation throughout my body. As I was flying over the countryside, I noticed people down below. With my eagle eyes I recognised the people. They were people that had hurt me in the past. And I had the realisation that they had not intentionally hurt me, that it was a by-product of their own drama. I felt a flood of compassion toward them coming from my heart. My chest was warm and open. Then I saw myself among these people and realised that I too was fallible and made mistakes. I was not perfect. I felt a flood of compassion toward myself and forgave myself. It felt so much more real than any dream I have experienced. I know I was awake. And, more importantly, that feeling of compassion toward others has not left me. That experience changed my attitude to life and as a result has changed my life itself.

I have had many sessions since. Most are nowhere near as dramatic. Sometimes I just sleep. But always feel refreshed, better than an eight-hour sleep. And my mind is much sharper afterward.

As I say, I started acupuncture in 1998 and was treating patients for a wide variety of problems but mostly chronic pain, especially chronic non-specific lower back pain. Following Mikio Sankey's workshops in Melbourne, I came back wondering who I would try his style of acupuncture on. Most of my patients were not into meditation and I felt uncomfortable 'selling' the spiritual aspect of acupuncture. Then one day I performed this style of acupuncture on a regular acupuncture patient with lower back pain. I wondered if by altering a person's mental state with acupuncture would change their physical condition. After the treatment, the patient asked me what I had done differently as it seemed to him to be a lot more powerful in its effect. After treating him with this style for a few visits, he didn't need to come again as his lower back pain was dramatically better. That had been after I had treated him for several months with the regular Chinese style of acupuncture. I began exploring this idea more and more and got more powerful results with patients. Within three or four months I had changed most of my patients over to this style of acupuncture. I had learned Mikio's method, but gradually systematised, developed and adapted it to treat various medical problems. I regularly had patients remarking how they generally felt really well, that they were handling problems better at work and had stopped having arguments at home, but I didn't take much more notice than that.

All that changed about a year later. One patient, a 60-year-old woman had been attending the practice for about six years. She had widespread osteoarthritis affecting her hips, knees, hands and feet. She had total knee replacements in 2007 and 2009. I had been giving her regular TCM-based acupuncture from 2006 until the second knee replacement in 2009.

In 2011, she wanted to restart acupuncture for lymphoedema in her legs. After a few visits of not getting anywhere with TCM-based acupuncture, I changed to performing the new style of acupuncture. Very soon she reported that not only was she was getting better relief of the tight feeling in her legs, but also was getting relief of pain in her arthritic fingers and even her knees felt better. After a few more visits she was able to stop taking Doloxene 100 (dextropropoxyphene), a rather strong painkiller that she had been taking regularly since first attending the practice in 2005. Her last prescription was in December 2011. She has not taken any painkillers since.

She continued to come in about once a month for acupuncture, and after a while she asked whether, since she was feeling so well, she could come off her antidepressant, Zoloft 100 (sertraline). She had been taking this daily for sixteen years. Another doctor in the practice had tried reducing her to 50mg daily in 2010, but this was unsuccessful. I assessed her symptoms using a DASS questionnaire. DASS stands for Depression Anxiety Stress Scale and is a validated tool for measuring the degree of symptoms. Her score was 3–0–3 (that is, 3 for depression, 0 for anxiety and 3 for stress out of a maximum score of 21–21–21) which was within normal range. See Chapter 7: What is a DASS? for a more in-depth description of DASS questionnaires. I agreed to reduce her dose to 50mg daily. After eight weeks she was still well and happy, so I agreed to reduce to ½ a 50mg tablet, and then to taking a ½ tablet on alternate days after another eight weeks. After another four weeks of taking only 25mg of Zoloft every other day she reported being still well and happy and commented that she felt more teary watching sad movies and cried tears of joy at hearing Christmas carols the night before I saw her. She was feeling the full range of her emotions again. She said she felt happier than at any time in the last twenty years. I agreed to stop the antidepressant.

That was on 30 November 2013. She has not been on anti-depressants since. She has not required any further painkillers either, except when she broke her arm the following year. I hasten to add that because she was a pensioner she could only afford to come in for acupuncture about once a month during all that time. Also, earlier in her treatment I was doing much shorter treatments on her. I had been modifying the acupuncture as I went. The last dozen treatments had a much more powerful effect on her compared with what I was doing on her when she first started coming for acupuncture. And apart from breaking her arm she has not required acupuncture since. She still comes to the practice for a regular check-up, but is not on any regular medications and remains mobile, happy and cheerful.

I had been regularly telling my (doctor) wife about my successes with the acupuncture, but when I told her this story she insisted that I do a study. She had studied medicine more recently than me and was right into evidence-based medicine. 'Prove it!' she kept saying. Being a typical male, I said that I didn't need to prove that it worked because already I knew and so did my patients! How foolish was I? Anyway, she kept throwing 'Prove it!' at me whenever I told her another success story. It took another two years of this, but I finally got the message.

It seems obvious in hindsight (well to me anyway), that the scientific method begins with an observation. In this case, that a patient was able to come off an antidepressant after sixteen years. That led to (my wife, not me) questioning what was going on there. At the time there was no real evidence in the literature that acupuncture helped depression.

Following the scientific method, that led to a hypothesis: that the improvement in her mood was due to the acupuncture. From March 2016, I performed an observational study by following a few acupuncture patients with mental health problems and monitored their DASS results. I did that to see what happened – and to stop my wife nagging me. The results surprised not only her, but me as well. They can be found in Chapter 8: Case Studies if you really cannot wait to find out what happened.

But before looking at those cases, I would like to discuss the modern medical view of mental health disorders, and depression in particular, and the medical approach to treatment.

3

WHAT IS DEPRESSION?

LET'S START WITH WHAT DEPRESSION IS NOT

What is depression? That is a good question. In attempting to define depression, let me first say what depression is not. Depression is *not* a disease. It is not a disease, unlike say hepatitis. Depression is a mental disorder. I'll repeat that again. Depression is defined as a disorder not a disease. That is why the medical condition is called 'major depressive disorder' by doctors.

This is easy to overlook, both as a doctor and as a patient diagnosed with depression. The doctor doesn't look at people as a general population. The doctor deals with the person in front of them, the patient. Before a patient opens their mouth, their doctor is observing, looking for signs of illness. When the patient talks, the doctor listens for symptoms. The doctor interrogates, examines and, if necessary, orders tests to be done. The doctor is searching for patterns, patterns of symptoms and signs that fit in a category. Generally, these patterns are labelled diseases or syndromes. The reason we do this is so the doctor will know how to manage the patient and know what the most effective drug or surgical procedure is to fix the disease. If the doctor cannot fix it, at least he or she will know what to do to ameliorate the worst effects of the disease. The doctor can give advice and a prognosis, that is to say what the course of disease is likely to be.

For example, I walk out to the waiting room and call for Bill Jones (not his real name). He is a patient I have looked after for many years. Immediately, I notice that he doesn't look well. There is none of the usual spring in his step. He is not dressed in his usual business suit; he is wearing a t-shirt and tracksuit pants. As I greet him, I notice the beads of sweat, accompanied by a stale odour, together with matted hair. Most of all, I notice the jaundiced sclera. The whites of the eye are no longer white, but yellow. Before we sit down in my consulting room, I already have a fair idea of the diagnosis. I may be influenced knowing his age, social background and past medical history.

With a few questions and a medical examination, pathology testing and imaging will give me a confirmed diagnosis within a few hours. Knowing the diagnosis, whether it be Hepatitis A, B or C, or another hepatic cause such gallstones blocking the bile duct or metastases in the liver, I can formulate a plan of action for Bill and outline his prognosis. I know this because these diseases are well classified and taught in medical school. I know which drugs are appropriate for Bill, because the trials have been run on groups of patients with the various categories of hepatitis to prove what works and what doesn't. Physiologically, the systems in the human body behave in a similar way in all humans. This makes it easier to predict the course of an illness. Obviously, there is individual variation, and age and sex may play their part, but usually the variation is within a range. Hepatitis A will usually run its course within one to three weeks and will need no specific treatment. Whereas Hepatitis C will be lifelong unless treated with anti-viral drugs. My advice for Bill will be tailored to the specific virus that he has caught. In some instances, further investigation could be ordered. We may even need to refer him for a liver biopsy in certain circumstances. The histological report will give us information that cannot be found by any other method of investigation. When dealing with examples of patients like Bill, we can practise with a good degree of confidence.

There are no such obvious noticeable changes in the case of a mental illness such as depression. There are no symptoms or signs characteristic of depression. This may sound shocking to you, but there is no specific symptom the patient could indicate to us or sign we could find on examination that beyond a shadow of a doubt would give the diagnosis of major depressive disorder. There is no x-ray or blood test that your doctor could perform to confirm the diagnosis. So, what is to be done? How does the doctor come up with a diagnosis of major depressive disorder? Does the doctor guess?

HOW IS DEPRESSION CLASSIFIED? WHY BOTHER?

Ever since Adam named all the animals brought to him (Gen 2.9–10) man loves to classify things. It helps to bring about a sense of order, which leads to understanding and control. I have seen this with HIV/AIDS in the early 80s, and now with COVID-19. Initially there seems to be chaos, fear and uncertainty. The story of bringing these diseases under control starts with finding the pathogen and seeing where the virus fits into the phylogenetic tree of all life on Earth. Symptoms and signs are observed for the disease's patterns and complications. Various treatments are tried in controlled settings, and the medical world doesn't rest until control over the disease is attained.

This is what the medical world has tried to do with depression – and all mental illness for that matter. This has great advantages, but also brings about great disadvantages.

Classification of mental illness is not a recent phenomenon. The first real attempt at classifying mental illness was by Hippocrates

(c. 460–370 BCE), but our current systems have been developed since World War II. The first real attempt was with the sixth revision of the *International Classification of Diseases* (ICD-6), published by WHO in 1949. Interestingly, none of the previous five editions attempted to classify mental illness.

The section of ICD-6 classifying mental illness was widely ignored by every member of the United Nations. Every country followed their own system of diagnosis.[19]

In 1952 the American Psychiatric Association published the first edition of the *Diagnostic and Statistical Manual of Mental Disorders* (DSM-I). Though only listing 106 mental disorders in a small, 132-page paperback, it was found to be more useful than the ICD-6.

Since then the DSM has undergone a number of editions and revisions:

Edition	Publication Date	Number of Pages	Number of Diagnoses
DSM-I	1952	132	128
DSM-II	1968	119	193
DSM-III	1980	494	228
DSM-III-R	1987	567	253
DSM-IV	1994	886	383
DSM-IV-TR	2000	943	383
DSM-5	2013	947	541

Source: Diagnostic and Statistical Manual of Mental Disorders

As you can see, with each edition it has become much more complex, as indicated by the number of pages and the number of mental disorders listed. Nowadays in Australia, doctors generally follow the DSM classification system in preference to the ICD, now in its eleventh edition.

The section describing depressive disorders (an umbrella term for depression) is itself 34 pages long in the latest edition, DSM-5. (The perceptive will notice in the table that the American Psychiatric Association has entered the computer age by moving away from Roman numerals. That allows for a DSM-5.1 update at some stage!)

The DSM-5 divides depressive disorders into eight categories. These are listed together with my simplistic explanation of them:

1. Disruptive mood dysregulation disorder – uncontrollable temper outbursts in (usually male) children starting at 6–10 years of age
2. Major depressive disorder (MDD) – the usual form of clinical depression we consider in this book
3. Persistent depressive disorder (dysthymia) – MDD that has gone on for more than two years
4. Premenstrual dysphoric disorder – PMS where emotional upset or irritability is the main symptom at that time of the cycle
5. Substance/medication induced depressive disorder – depression triggered by various legal and illegal drugs (see Medical Masquerades of Depression later in this chapter).
6. Depressive disorder due to another medical condition – depression caused by illness (again, see Medical Masquerades of Depression later in this chapter).
7. Other specified depressive disorder – the patient has had symptoms for less than two weeks or doesn't have enough symptoms to fit the diagnosis of MDD
8. Unspecified depressive disorder – the doctor thinks the patient is depressed but doesn't have the time or ability to make a full assessment (e.g. in an emergency room).

So, just because a patient is clinically depressed doesn't necessarily mean they have major depressive disorder.

This situation is further complicated because any of these depressive disorders may be qualified with the following modifiers:

1. With anxious distress – depression with anxiety, or anxiety with depression
2. With mixed features – some degree of mania (elevated, expansive mood and activity)
3. With melancholic features – profoundly despondent, complete loss of pleasure, lost interest in eating (think 'Ode on Melancholy' by John Keats)
4. With atypical features – weight gain, sleepiness, yet cheers up in some situations
5. With psychotic features – hallucinations, delusions
6. With catatonia – slowed down almost to a complete halt*
7. With peripartum onset – generally known as post-natal depression, but can begin before delivery
8. With seasonal pattern – usually occurring in winter and getting better in spring.

The DSM-5 then states that the disorder be specified by current severity:

- Mild
- Moderate
- Severe.

And then finally specify if it is:

- In partial remission
- In full remission.

By labelling the person as in full remission, the implication is that a person is never really rid of depression. Even if they feel and act normal, it is lurking in the background ready to pounce when the patient's guard is down. This is often why a doctor will tell you that you need the antidepressant for life, even though you feel you have recovered from the depression.

Obviously, the combinations and permutations are huge. In the above list there is potential for every person who ever felt depressed to be given a diagnosis – and, if not, they probably have an unspecified depressive disorder (tongue only slightly in cheek).

DIAGNOSIS OF MAJOR DEPRESSIVE DISORDER

Let us focus on major depressive disorder, which is the main form of clinical depression. The following is the diagnostic criteria of major depressive episodes taken from the DSM-5.

DIAGNOSTIC CRITERIA OF MAJOR DEPRESSIVE EPISODES

A. Five (or more) of the following symptoms have been present during the same 2-week period and represent a change from previous functioning; at least one of the symptoms is either (1) depressed mood or (2) loss of interest or pleasure. **Note:** Do not include symptoms that are clearly attributable to another medical condition.

1. Depressed mood most of the day, nearly every day, as indicated by either subjective report (e.g., the patient says they feel sad, empty, hopeless) or observation made by others (e.g., appears tearful). (**Note:** In children and adolescents, can be irritable mood.)

2. Markedly diminished interest or pleasure in all, or almost all, activities most of the day, nearly every day (as indicated by either subjective account or observation).

3. Significant weight loss when not dieting or weight gain (e.g. a change of more than 5 per cent of body weight in a month), or decrease or increase in appetite nearly every day. (Note: In children, consider failure to make expected weight gain.)

4. Insomnia or hypersomnia nearly every day.

5. Psychomotor agitation (fidgety) or retardation (slowed speech, decreased movement) nearly every day (observable by others, not merely subjective feelings of restlessness or being slowed down).

6. Fatigue or loss of energy nearly every day.

7. Feelings of worthlessness, or excessive or inappropriate guilt (which may be delusional) nearly every day (not merely self-reproach or guilt about being sick).

8. Diminished ability to think or concentrate, or indecisiveness, nearly every day (either by subjective account or as observed by others).

9. Recurrent thoughts of death (not just fear of dying), recurrent suicidal ideation without a specific plan, or a suicide attempt or a specific plan for committing suicide.

As you can see, it sounds very precise. The diagnosis seems clear cut at first glance. If a person has symptom 1 and 2, you only have to find three more symptoms out of the remaining seven. If they have had the symptoms for fourteen days or more, voilà: you have your diagnosis. Is it that straight forward? No. As the authors of the *Diagnostic and Statistical Manual of Mental Disorders* themselves say in the introduction to the fifth edition, 'Clinical training and experience are needed to use DSM for determining a diagnosis.' In other words, the DSM is not to be used by armchair amateurs using a tick-all-the-boxes approach to diagnosis, but by those who have been trained and have sufficient experience of dealing with patients with mental health issues.

The authors go on to say that diagnostic criteria '*require clinical expertise to differentiate from normal life variation and transient response to stress*'. So clinical experience is required not only to differentiate the symptoms and signs of one mental disorder from another, but to even differentiate a mental disorder from a normal, mentally healthy response to a given situation.

'In short, we have come to recognize that the boundaries between disorders are more porous than originally perceived.' (AMERICAN PSYCHIATRIC ASSOCIATION, 2013)

So, this classification system is a guide to making a diagnosis of a mental disorder. The boundaries between depression and bipolar are not fixed, unlike the species boundaries between a cat and a dog.

Depression refers to an emotional state in which the person feels down or sad. We all know what it feels like to feel down or sad at times. As the DSM authors state, these feelings can be 'normal life variation' or a 'transient response to stress'.

If the depressed feeling is prolonged, this is a depressed mood. If the depressed mood becomes a habit and continues for more than a couple of weeks, it *may* be considered a clinical depression. So, what makes depression clinical depression? What makes depression an illness is the extent of the feeling, both in time and degree.

The DSM-5 refers to clinical depression as being 'a disorder', and not a disease. And note that the manual is not called the 'Diagnostic and Statistical Manual of Mental *Diseases*'. In fact, the manual classifies *all* mental illness as disorders. For a full discussion of the significance of this, please see my first book, *Stick it to Depression: Another Tool in Your Doctor's Bag*. But suffice it to say, there is a world of difference between a disorder where the thoughts, emotion and behaviour may be hard to distinguish from normal to that of a disease. The following example can give you an idea of what I mean.

WOULD YOU FEEL HAPPY IF YOUR PARTNER DIED A MONTH AGO?

What are you talking about Dr Alex? I feel lost and lonely. I wake up and remember my partner has gone. Friends comfort me and cheer me up, but there's not a day when I don't miss my partner. We've been together since high school, you know.

You seemed depressed to me.

Sure, I feel so down. I toss and turn half the night. I've even lost interest in going to the pub with my mates.

Let me prescribe for you the latest SSRI, Happizac. It will make you feel happy again.

Great. Thanks, doc.

This is not such a far-fetched conversation. In fact, doctors are basically encouraged to think this way.

When I was a hospital resident, bereavement over a loved one was considered a normal and dramatic shift in one's life. The then-current manual, the DSM-III, stated that a doctor should not diagnose depression within *two years* of losing someone close. I remember the elderly Greek women in my extended family would in fact wear black for the rest of their lives after losing their husbands.

In 1994 the DSM-IV was published. They reduced the bereavement exclusion period to two *months*.

The latest edition, DSM-5, has reduced that period to *two weeks*. Yes, you read that correctly.

In one generation, the bereavement period has shortened from two years to two weeks. We truly live in a nanosecond world, where we are not given the luxury of time to mourn.

US figures demonstrate that around 1990, 3 per cent of over-65s were on antidepressants. The latest figures show 19 per cent of over-65s are taking antidepressants.

Here is another example of so-called disease-mongering, where the boundaries of illness are widened and then the condition promoted as being treatable:

The DSM-5 defines the diagnosis of social anxiety disorder, formerly known as 'social phobia'. in my younger days it was known as 'being shy'. The DSM-5 defines social anxiety disorder as being when 'the individual is fearful or anxious about or avoidant of social interactions and situations that involve the possibility of being scrutinised'. I think you will agree that this a broad definition. Most people would be quite relaxed talking to a group of their friends, but I am sure that a large proportion of people would feel extremely anxious if asked to give a speech in front of a stadium full of people.

Does this mean all these people have a mental disorder? I think not. Yet statistically, 11 per cent of the Australian people experience this condition in their lifetime, according to Beyond Blue.[20]

That is a lot of people. Needless to say, the drug companies heavily promote to doctors that SSRI and SNRI are an effective treatment for social anxiety disorder.

A SIMPLER CLASSIFICATION OF DEPRESSIVE DISORDERS

When I went through medical school, mental disorders were broadly categorised into psychotic and neurotic disorders. The term 'psychotic disorders' is still favoured by the medical profession. Whereas 'neurotic disorders' is not.

In relation to depression, psychotic disorders included manic depressive psychosis, now known as bipolar disorder, and severe depression with features of psychosis. Patients with psychosis showed symptoms that were difficult for normal people to relate to, such as hallucinations, flights of ideas and extreme grandiose ideas.

I was taught that neurotic patients experience symptoms that we all experience from time to time such as anxiety and feeling depressed, only more extreme or more constant. The majority of people with depressive disorders and anxiety disorders fit into this category formerly called 'neurotic'.

I was taught that if there were no psychotic features, depression was either endogenous or reactive. Endogenous depression, or now known as melancholic depression, comprises around 10 per cent of patients with depression, is thought to be due to biologically based and more severe, and will generally require drug treatment and probably will require the help of psychiatrists.

Reactive, or now referred to as non-melancholic depression, relates to the fact that external factors that have triggered the depression in a person who has previously been generally mentally well, but then find themselves not coping with a life stressor. This kind of depression commonly presents in the mild to moderate range. These are the people who are relatively easily treated by non-drug methods and are the people that I am focusing on in this book. The good news is that these comprise 90 per cent of patients presenting with symptoms of depression.[21] Even today the Black Dog Institute finds that categorising depression into the melancholic form and the non-melancholic form useful.[22]

So then, what is depression (of the non-melancholic variety)? In Western medicine, doctors use diagnostic tools like the criteria discussed earlier to try to apply a tick-box approach to a problem that is by its very nature constantly shifting to fit the patient into a category. There is a tendency to label a patient as having depression and then go immediately to an antidepressant to 'fix' the depression, so to speak, just as a doctor would diagnose pneumonia and immediately treat it with antibiotics. The doctor may add counselling as an adjunct, just as the doctor may add oxygen or physiotherapy as an adjunct to antibiotics. But doctors' primary training is still focused on treating the depression with drugs, antidepressants. Just as you would call on a plumber to fix a blocked drain or a surgeon to cut out a diseased gallbladder, call on a doctor if you want drug treatment.

I think the reality is that 'depression' is no more a diagnosis than 'cough'. I would argue that depression is a symptom and not a disorder. When looking at depression in this way, the obvious question that arises in my mind is what is this a symptom of? That is, what is the underlying cause?

When treating depression as a *symptom* it changes the dynamics of the whole consultation. I explain that depression is a symptom, a warning from their subconscious mind that things aren't going well for them. They shouldn't dismiss it or try to suppress it but address it. When the patient sees the depression as a call to action, a signal that they need to make changes in their life, the patient becomes empowered. By just saying, 'The serotonin levels in your brain are low. This pill will elevate those levels,' we run the risk of disempowering our patients, turning them into dependent victims.

If we ask the patient for their understanding of why they think they are depressed, they sometimes know the reason. It may be an obvious trigger such as a relationship breakup, an act of infidelity or a diagnosis of cancer. I would think most general practitioners would be alert to this and immediately counsel the patient or refer them to a psychologist so that the patient feels understood, heard and given strategies to deal with the situation. In a large percentage of such cases, antidepressants are not necessary.

However, in my experience, a lot of patients can't identify a specific incident or situation as a cause or trigger of the depression and blame it on 'everyone in my family has depression', 'my life is crap' or 'I have a chemical imbalance in my brain'. It is easy to agree with the patient and treat them with antidepressants. But there is an effective alternative as I will discuss in this book.

THE DANGERS OF PIGEONHOLING

There are obvious advantages to a classification system such as the DSM. It gives doctors a framework to understand what mental problems patients are dealing with and helps us explain to them what is going on. It enables us to compare the effects of various treatments in trials on groups of people fitting within the one category. It gives some predictive value, so that we can let the patient know what to expect in terms of the natural progression of the condition and what treatments are likely to work.

But there are obvious dangers too. The idea of pigeonholing is to classify disparate items into a limited number of categories; that is, to sort things into groups of like items. In our practice we still have a cabinet on the wall of our administration room. It is designed as a set of boxes that are open at the front and each one is labelled with the name of each of the doctors in the practice. Our office junior collects the mail from the post office each day and brings back the pile of mail. It is a simple process to read the name of the doctor on the envelope and put it into the appropriate pigeonhole. That way, the mail is sorted efficiently once instead of each doctor rummaging through a pile of mail on the desk and making a mess in the process.

Human beings aren't really like a pile of mail though. Sure, some mental symptoms and signs are relatively clear-cut and easy to classify, such as auditory or visual hallucinations, but others are vague and more open to interpretation, such as a person's ability to maintain eye contact or how loud or fast they speak. One doctor will emphasise some symptoms or signs while another will place emphasis on different symptoms or signs. Patients themselves will emphasise different symptoms on different days, depending on how they feel.

Psychiatrists are human too and want to classify the patients they study and help by emulating the classification used for physical disease states. A system to classify the thoughts, feelings and behaviour of humans is inherently imperfect and messy. That is why with each edition of the DSM things are becoming more complicated, and something like the depressive disorders have many qualifications. Trying to define a disorder by saying that the patient must fit an arbitrary five criteria out of nine adds to the complications and murkiness. Diagnosing is an art as much as it is a science.

By comparison, physicists and chemists studying the elements have made a definitive pigeonhole system called the periodic table of elements. There are 92 naturally occurring elements and a further 26 artificially created elements. So, the periodic table has 118 pigeonholes. Copper is number 29 and zinc is number 30. No scientist would mistake one for the other. An atom could be zinc or it could be copper, but not both. Whereas a human could be zinc one day, copper the next, or have qualities of both simultaneously. Then on the next visit present as something completely different, like uranium!

When I graduated in 1979 there were 193 pigeonholes you could stick people with mental illness in, whereas today there are 541 pigeonholes to choose from. As the authors of the DSM admit, there is no fixed boundary between depression and anxiety, let alone between the various depressive disorders, or for that matter between clinical depression and a mentally well person experiencing a depressed feeling.

Sometimes the depressive symptoms dominate, and other days the anxiety. Does the patient have recent onset of major depressive disorder with anxious distress or does the patient with generalised anxiety disorder have recent onset of a depressive disorder? Or do they have adjustment disorder with mixed anxiety and depressed mood? Possibly it may be post-traumatic stress disorder, where the patient hasn't made the connection between a past traumatic event and their current depressed mood. Or maybe they really have bipolar II disorder with a major depressive episode, though their hypomanic features lasted only three days and not the four days minimum required for a diagnosis. Or maybe they are within the spectrum of 'normal'.

A number of years ago my dad was complaining to his GP about all his problems, and his GP wanted to prescribe him anti-depressants as a result. My dad was shocked. 'Whatever for?' he asked. 'I'm not depressed. This is how I always am!'

Psychiatrists and psychologists are only human. With each new edition of the DSM there a host of new fashionable diagnoses to try out on their patients. Patients are moved from one pigeonhole to another. Some people who previously didn't fit well into any pigeonhole may now have a pigeonhole ready made for them. In my career, I have witnessed six of the seven editions and revisions of the DSM. With each edition there is a host of new diagnoses and a whole range of human behaviour that will now fit into a pigeonhole.

A classic example of a pigeonhole with an ever-rising rate of diagnosis and increasing use of (overuse, in my opinion) medication is attention deficit hyperactivity disorder (ADHD). In 1968 the DSM-II was released with a new pigeonhole, a new diagnosis in children: hyperkinetic reaction of childhood.[23]

At the time, the condition was considered fairly uncommon. Little mention was made of it when I was in medical school in the 1970s. I think I recall it being briefly discussed in one lecture, lumped in with other then uncommon childhood conditions like autism. I don't think that it is a coincidence that in the same year, 1968, the US National Institute of Mental Health (NIMH) issued grants to researchers to study the effects of stimulants (dexamphetamine and methylphenidate) on children with this condition. In 1980 the DSM-III changed the name of this condition to attention deficit disorder, with or without hyperactivity.

I started general practice in 1982 and found that by the mid-1980s parents were starting to bring their children (mostly sons) in to see me, having been advised by their teachers that they were to be checked for this disorder. I usually observed children sitting in my rooms wanting to touch everything not bolted down, and parents generally ignoring this behaviour but often insisting on a referral to a specialist. My own thoughts were that healthy boys were often fidgety – it was just boys being kept in a classroom who were perhaps better wired for playing outdoors on a sunny day than sitting still listening to someone talking to them. However, often specialists would prescribe stimulants, which meant that over time these kids were being medicated to calm them down a bit. Ironically, it was also proposed by some specialists back in those times that these children were okay to go off their medication during the summer holidays as school was out and they were freer to roam and play.

In the 1980s and 90s a seeming epidemic ensued of teachers wanting to have calm kids in the classroom and parents wanting to please the teachers. Call me cynical, but that was how it often seemed to me and was borne out in many conversations with other GPs at that time.

I have a relative who is on this medication for ADHD (the name was changed yet again in DSM-III-R –the 'R' is for 'revised' – in 1987). Yet I have seen him sitting still, playing on the PlayStation for hours on end fully attentive to the game, whether he is on medication or not.

The DSM-5 refers to ADHD as 'a neurodevelopmental disorder'. It sounds as though they are stating that something has gone wrong with the development of the brain. However, they are not. Merely that the condition 'manifests in the developmental period', commonly called 'childhood'. Nevertheless, the implication that something has gone wrong in the brain is still there. I wonder how many doctors, let alone parents and teachers, would understand the subtle distinction.

The diagnosing of children continues unabated. See, for example, the Centers for Disease Control and Prevention (CDC) website.[24]

The trend of the following graph found there is very clear.

ADHD DIAGNOSIS THROUGHOUT THE YEARS: ESTIMATES FROM PUBLISHED
NATIONALLY REPRESENTATIVE SURVEY DATA
(Percent of children with a parent-reported ADHD diagnosis)

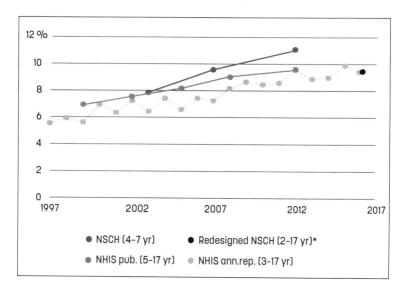

The number of children diagnosed with ADHD has virtually doubled in the twenty-year period to 2017. Currently around 10 per cent of children in the US have been diagnosed with ADHD.

Interestingly, states on the eastern seaboard of the US have a diagnosis rate two to three times that of those states in the west. The application of the diagnostic criteria doesn't sound very objective to me.

The most recent figures for Australia, also from 2011, showed that between 2002 and 2009 the growth in prescriptions for stimulants was 87 per cent. It is not called the health industry for nothing![25]

A recent study reported in the *Medical Journal of Australia*, seems to confirm the danger of pigeonholing mental disorders.[26] In analysing the prescribing of stimulants for ADHD in 311,384 Western Australian schoolchildren, they found the very worrying figure that the youngest children (born in June) in any class were *twice* as likely to be diagnosed with ADHD than the oldest (born in July the previous year). Their immaturity is being mistaken for a mental disorder. This should shock us.

Further, a 2010 Western Australia Department of Health study found ADHD-diagnosed children who had used stimulants were 10.5 times *more* likely to fail academically than children diagnosed with ADHD but never medicated. So much for medication helping their attention deficit, and so much for evidence-based medicine. It is now nine years later, but I don't hear cries from doctors to stop prescribing these drugs for our most vulnerable population.[27]

If all the above doesn't outrage you, the DSM-III-R brought out the category oppositional defiant disorder (ODD). These are children who 'often lose temper, often touchy, easily annoyed and often angry or resentful'. Worse, 'they often argue with authority figures'. I kid you not. This is found in the diagnostic criteria, on p. 462 of the DSM-5. I am reminded of one young teenage patient with this diagnosis. She was very intelligent and her mother had a much more modest intelligence. The girl had a smart mouth and always out-argued her mother. Personally, I silently sided with the girl. Estimates of the number of children with this 'condition' vary, but I have seen figures of up to 20 per cent. At present, no drug therapy is indicated, but how long before drug trials are run? How many editions of the DSM will come out before virtually every child on the planet will fit in a pigeonhole?

I know that I have taken a bit of a detour from discussing depression, but firstly I thought it important to highlight the dangers of pigeonholing in our most vulnerable group, our children.

Secondly, around 60 per cent of children with ADHD become adults with ADHD. And around 50 per cent of these adults also have anxiety, and a large percentage of the rest have depression, bipolar disorder or other mental illness.[28]

Personally, I have used low level laser acupuncture (that has no known side effects) on a handful of children with ADHD, and another 'neurodevelopmental' disorder Asperger's Syndrome, and they usually become much more focused and calmer after only a handful of sessions. I would love to able to do an acupuncture clinical trial on these kids.

THE DANGERS OF MULTIPLE DIAGNOSES

Another example of the dangers of pigeonholing is a patient being given multiple diagnoses over time. This is partly due to fashion and changing definitions from the DSM, partly due to a difference of opinion between various doctors and psychologists that a patient presents to and partly due to the changing presentation of symptoms that a patient has. One of the worse cases I have seen is a patient of mine, we'll call her Betty. She is 82 years old and has been given various diagnoses over the years. Betty has a background of a difficult childhood, being a victim of physical and emotional abuse by her mother, then as an adult, abuse by her alcoholic husband and, most recently, emotional abuse by her adult daughter. She was diagnosed as having depression in 1976. Coinciding with the release of the DSM-III in 1980 she was diagnosed with the then-new condition post-traumatic stress disorder, which I think was a fair call. She has been a patient of our practice for the past twelve years and during that time has seen sixteen GPs here, though she has usually seen me for her mental health problems over the past nine years. Just before I started seeing her regularly, she saw a psychologist in late 2010. Betty was assessed according to criteria of the DSM-IV-TR ('text revision', in case you were wondering) and was diagnosed with (and I quote):

1. Major depressive disorder – recurrent, chronic
2. panic disorder without agoraphobia

3. generalised anxiety disorder
4. personality disorder not otherwise specified with borderline and paranoid features.

Betty never went back to that psychologist, and the psychologist she has been seeing ever since has never raised the possibility of diagnoses two, three or four. I asked Betty what happened with that first psychologist and she said that she disagreed with them about diagnoses two and three. She said that she never had panic attacks, and wasn't overly anxious and worrying about her health, family and finances. Because she argued and disagreed with the psychologist about the diagnoses and planned treatment, the psychologist said that she was being paranoid and slapped on the final diagnosis!

Betty had been on various antidepressants for many years and had been taking Lexapro (escitalopram) for the last four years before seeing me. She was referred to me by another doctor in our practice for Transformational Acupuncture to relieve the stress and tension in her neck and shoulders. She found that it not only relieved the muscular tension but also helped her mood. So much so, that after a couple of years she stopped her antidepressant. That was in 2012. I have been seeing her for acupuncture monthly since, and she sees a psychologist at our practice, also monthly. We have helped her through a number of family crises including the death of her husband, abusive episodes from her 50-year-old daughter and dealing with her husband's will and sale of property. I think giving Betty the skills to deal with life's circumstances is much more empowering for her and being there for her through the tougher times has made a big difference. Through the last seven years she hasn't felt the need for medication, just acupuncture and regular counselling sessions with the psychologist. I have never seen any evidence of excessive anxiety or panic attacks and she has never displayed any paranoia or personality disorder.

MEDICAL MASQUERADES OF DEPRESSION

In considering the cause of depression it is important to rule out a number of medical conditions first. Particularly in this age of Dr Google, patients may feel depressed, look to herbs or natural therapies for depression and then go ahead treat themselves, not realising they may have a physical explanation for feeling depressed. It is important to treat these conditions optimally to reduce the risk of this happening. This list includes:

- hypothyroidism
- coeliac disease
- iron deficiency
- poorly controlled diabetes
- coronary heart disease
- chronic kidney disease
- auto-immune diseases including Lupus
- neurological diseases such as multiple sclerosis, Parkinson's Disease, Strokes
- chronic pain
- substance and alcohol abuse
- and even post-viral conditions.

I was reminded of this during the last flu season, when for three or four weeks after the symptoms of fever, cough, achy joints and congested head had resolved, I still felt lethargic, sleeping long hours and feeling down. I had no motivation to return to work. Fortunately, my doctor-wife was aware that this was purely a physical response to the illness, and not just being lazy and feeling sorry for myself. It made me more sympathetic to those who suffer post-viral fatigue following Ross River virus, Barmah Forest virus, glandular fever, HIV/AIDS and many other viral infections that can leave people feeling depleted and depressed for a long time.

In fact, I often see patients with chronic fatigue syndrome who have been prescribed antidepressants. In situations like this, the line blurs between the illness causing the depression and the depression developing as a response to how the person feels about having a chronic debilitating illness.

Medications can be less obvious causes of depression. It is important to make sure that other medication you are already taking is not causing or contributing to the depression. These include a group of drugs known as beta blockers. Before ACE inhibitors became available in the 1980s, beta blockers were the most popular blood pressure medications and are still widely used today, such as propranolol (Inderal), metoprolol (Betaloc, Minax) and atenolol (Tenormin, Noten). One of the marketing strategies of ACE inhibitor drug reps in the early days was promoting that their drugs not only lowered blood pressure but actually made patients feel happy and experience 'joie de vivre'. I was encouraged to try switching my hypertensive patients onto their drugs. And I found it to be true! A lot of them reported that they slept better and that their nightmares even disappeared. Marvellous! The truth became apparent though that it wasn't a result of the new drug, but taking the patients off their beta blockers!

Other drugs that can cause depression include the combined contraceptive pill; statins used to lower cholesterol; corticosteroids such as prednisone used in autoimmune diseases; and proton pump inhibitors and H2 antagonists used for reflux and indigestion. Given the sheer number of people on these medications and that they are not necessarily recognised by patients as possibly being a cause of depression, a massive number of people could be unnecessarily depressed. If you think that your depression may be linked to a medication you are taking, I urge you to discuss this with your medical practitioner. I hasten to caution anyone to not stop their medication without medical advice.

It is also important to note that any of the psychoactive drugs can cause a depressed feeling, ironically including antidepressants themselves. Even to the point of increasing the risk of suicide. This is why it is especially important to monitor a severely depressed person for the first few weeks of commencing antidepressants. A colleague of mine commenced a depressed teenage patient on antidepressants and received a call only three or four days later from his school to say that the teen had climbed onto the roof of the school gym and had to be talked down. This was an individual who had never displayed any signs of wanting to self-harm.

The benzodiazepines, like Valium (diazepam) can certainly reduce anxiety, but did you know, they can cause a depressed mood too? If a person takes them long term they are at an increased risk of chronic depression.

Many years ago, in the 1980s, I had minor procedure and that night I was offered a Mogadon (nitrazepam) 5mg tablet to help me sleep. When I awoke the next morning I felt so groggy and depressed I couldn't believe it. The operation was a complete success and I was discharged, but I felt so miserable. I felt so dead inside. I just wanted to cry. Fortunately, the feeling wore off a few hours later. I've never had one since. That experience certainly changed my prescribing habits, I can tell you. 'Moggies' were quite popular with little old ladies in those days, but I can't remember when I last prescribed it.

Benzodiazepines are often prescribed in the early stages of depression, if the patient has significant anxiety or is unable to sleep. It is important to monitor for worsening of depressive symptoms due to the drug itself.

This brings me to the subject of modern medicine's solution to the problem of depression.

4

THE SOLUTION: PILLS, PILLS, PILLS

THE RISE AND RISE OF SSRIS

In our present society the idea of taking pills doesn't have to be sold. Generally, when a patient attends a doctor, the expectation is that they will leave the clinic with a prescription. To my recollection, I have never attended a medical education evening sponsored by a pharmaceutical company where the focus wasn't on a drug as a solution to a particular medical problem. For example, before statins came on the market in the late 1980s, I cannot recall cholesterol being the subject at any pharmaceutical company sponsored event. It was all about treating hypertension with the latest beta blocker, then the latest ACE inhibitor followed by the latest ARB. For the next few years after, it seemed that treating cholesterol with statins was the subject at every other event, and why Brand A was a better statin than Brand B. Similarly, with selective serotonin reuptake inhibitors, SSRIs, in treating depression. I can't recall non-pharmacological treatment of depression as the subject at any pharmaceutical company sponsored event. In fact, I don't think there were any pharmaceutical company sponsored events on depression before the arrival of Prozac, the first SSRI in Australia around 1990. At these events only lip service is paid to talking about lifestyle modification. It was all about the latest wonder drug.

Increasingly in the West, whatever the problem, people want a quick fix. Whether it is drive-through fast food, instant noodles, online food-ordering companies or one-click purchases from the comfort of your lounge, people expect things fast and with as little effort as possible on their part. We expect our gadgets to work first time, every time. If it stops working, throw it out. The new gadget will work faster, be bigger, or smaller, whatever. It's bound to be better than the now obsolete gadget. We try to treat our bodies the same way. If your knee wears out, get a replacement. If your kidneys fail, get a transplant. If your eye lens fails, get it replaced. I'm not saying this is wrong, but this is our expectation. 'It's your day, don't share it with a headache', was the old refrain from Vincent's. Take a painkiller and carry on as usual. If you feel depressed, take an antidepressant and carry on as usual.

The powerful 'brand you can trust' messaging from the health industry reinforces this notion of 'a pill for every ill'. The American Psychological Association quotes a study reported in the *Canadian Medical Association Journal* from 2003 that showed that depressed patients asking their doctor for an antidepressant by name were *17 times* more likely to walk out with a prescription than those who just described their symptoms.[29]

When I first entered medicine, tricyclics were the main anti-depressants in use. They were reserved for more severe depression and the main reason was the side effects, particularly a dry mouth, sleepiness and dizziness. Patients with mild or even moderate symptoms often couldn't tolerate these side effects. They made these patients feel worse rather than better. There were potentially more serious cardiac side effects that also had doctors concerned. So, these drugs were reserved for the more seriously depressed.

The newer agents, SSRIs and serotonin-norepinephrine (noradrenaline) reuptake inhibitors (SNRIs), don't have as severe or obvious side effects, though they do have significant side effects in a lot of people. So, over the years, the use of the antidepressants has been pushed into the moderate range of depression and even into mild depression – even though there is no conclusive evidence that antidepressants are effective in the mild to moderate range of depression. In fact, it has been suggested that 82 per cent of the effectiveness of antidepressants is due to the placebo effect.[30]

As well as being used in milder forms of depression, the use of antidepressants has been pushed in younger and younger patients. In the ten-year period from 2008 to 2018, the dispensing of anti-depressants to children, adolescents and young adults increased 66 per cent in Australia.[31]

Between 2006 and 2016, amongst 5–19 year olds in the states of New South Wales and Victoria there was a 98 per cent increase in intentional poisonings, and this was using the very medications prescribed to help them.[32] The authors concluded, 'there is clear evidence that more young Australians are taking antidepressants, and more young Australians are killing themselves and self-harming, often by intentionally overdosing on the very substances that are supposed to help them.' Antidepressants continue to be prescribed to children and adolescents despite the lack of evidence that antidepressants even work in children.[33]

EXAMPLES OF ANTIDEPRESSANTS

Class of drug	Generic name	Brand name
SSRIs (selective serotonin reuptake inhibitor)	fluoxetine	Prozac
	sertraline	Zoloft
	citalopram	Cipramil
	escitalopram	Lexapro
	paroxetine	Aropax
	fluvoxamine	Luvox
SNRIs (serotonin norepinephrine (noradrenaline) reuptake inhibitor)	venlafaxine	Effexor
	duloxetine	Cymbalta
	desvenlafaxine	Pristiq

TCAs	amitriptyline	Endep
(tricyclic antidepressant):	doxepin	Sinequan
much less	imipramine	Tofranil
commonly used	dothiepin	Dothep
nowadays	nortriptyline	Nortriptyline
	trimipramine	Surmontil

There are a number of other classes of antidepressants, but this above list accounts for the majority of prescriptions. Generic name = the scientific chemical name given to a drug – often a tongue-twister, e.g. desvenlafaxine. Brand name = the drug named by a specific company – usually easy to remember, e.g. Pristiq

In the last few years, antidepressants have been promoted for treating anxiety, social phobia (shyness, if you like) and panic disorder. So much so that Australia ranks third on the list of OECD countries for the consumption of antidepressants.

We may be the lucky country, but we are not the happy country. The numbers are mind-boggling. Given the wide promotion of antidepressants and lure of a quick fix, together with a culture that readily accepts that there is 'a pill for every ill', it is no wonder GPs are being overwhelmed with patients presenting with mental health issues. In 2000 over 4 per cent of the Australian population were taking antidepressants. By 2009 that number had doubled to 8 per cent. As of 2019, 12.5 per cent of Australians were on antidepressants, that's a full 3 million people, including over 100,000 children. And according to Pharmaceutical Benefits Scheme (PBS) statistics, general practitioners accounted for nearly 90 per cent of those prescriptions.[34]

It just beggars belief really, but a quarter of women in the United States in their forties and fifties are on antidepressants. And I'm sure Australia isn't far behind. I have met many female patients who have told me that they were advised to take antidepressants by their previous male doctor because they cried when they described their ongoing medical problems – whatever their illness! When I first listened to such stories, I thought the patients were exaggerating or just plain mistaken. But unfortunately, I have heard this again and again over the years. I can virtually guarantee that if you are a female attending a male doctor and cry while you tell him about your ongoing fatigue, tiredness or bad domestic life, you will be prescribed antidepressants. If not on the first visit, then the second or third. I would venture a guess that there would be a direct correlation between the frequency of visits to a male GP by a female complaining of these problems and the likelihood of being prescribed antidepressants. Males tend to want to fix things. It sits much better with the male psyche than 'just listening'. Men want to take action. I am not aware of any study comparing the prescribing habits of male doctors with female doctors, but I think it would be interesting.

TRUST ME, I'M A DRUG REP

In the 1960s and 70s many a celebrity overdosed on barbiturates and died. For example, Judy Garland, Jimi Hendrix, Marilyn Monroe and Dinah Washington. The barbiturates were prescribed for insomnia and from this perspective they worked well. Unfortunately, they also depressed the centre in the brain concerned with breathing. These people and many others died, whether intentional or not, because they literally stopped breathing in their sleep. Yet, when I was an intern in 1979, it was still common practice in the hospital to treat patients bed-ridden with severe sciatica using a cocktail of paracetamol, codeine and barbiturates in high doses.

Conveniently, the days were numbered for barbiturates only when alternative drugs were available. 'Now that safer benzodiazepines are available, why prescribe barbiturates any longer?' was a common refrain from drug reps at the time. 'They are non-addictive and safe to treat insomnia and anxiety, unlike the nasty barbiturates.'

When diazepam (Valium), the first benzodiazepine was marketed in 1963, it was considered a great step forward. By the time I became an intern in 1979, more than two billion tablets a year were being sold. It apparently cost US1c to manufacture each tablet. A great money spinner. But time has revealed the addictive nature of Valium.

The response of the pharmaceutical companies was to invent even more benzodiazepines. Through the 1980s alprazolam (Xanax), clobazam (Frisium), clonazepam (Rivotril) and fluni-trazepam (Rohypnol), were each marketed to me by drug reps as a suitable replacement, claiming they were less addictive than Valium. The use of all these drugs is now highly restricted in Australia because of their addictive nature.

In the 1990s along came SSRI antidepressant drugs, initially beginning with fluoxetine (Prozac). Prozac came to the world with rock-star status, even making it on the front cover of *Newsweek* as 'Prozac: A Breakthrough Drug for Depression'. Promotors such as Dr Peter Kramer, in his book *Listening to Prozac* in 1993, stated that it would make patients 'better than well'.

Initially, SSRI drugs were marketed for treatment of depression. With time, the use of them has broadened to treat anxiety conditions, such generalised anxiety disorder, panic disorder and obsessive compulsive disorder. Needless to say, the drug reps have insisted they are not addictive, unlike benzodiazepines. But what else do you call it where the patient becomes more anxious when they try to stop a drug used to treat anxiety? Let's call it 'discontinuation syndrome', not drug addiction.

Call me cynical, but I predict this situation will continue until the drug companies produce a new class of drug that 'aren't addictive, unlike those SSRIs'.

A SHOCKING SIDE EFFECT

Do you know what it is like to have an electric shock? I do. It's not pleasant. In my teenage years I was right into electronics. In those days, before integrated circuits, black and white televisions had valves in them. The valves looked a bit like old-fashioned light globes and used to blow about as often. One day, a valve in the power section of our TV died. The power section operates under high voltage. I'm not talking about a 9V battery instead of a 1.5V battery. I'm talking about 22,000V. My dad was a lecturer in electronics at a TAFE college. So naturally, I thought I knew a lot about electronics and knew which valve to replace. However, I didn't know enough to check that the power cord was removed from the wall before putting my hand inside the back of the TV. The back of my hand grazed against a 'live' panel. Bang. A numbing pain shot up my arm. The jolt made my hand spasm. Fortunately, the spasm threw my arm away from the back of the TV (thank God). It left my arm feeling numb for some minutes and my ego feeling bruised for a lot longer.

In my first ten years of general practice I never heard a patient complain of strange electric shock sensations in the body and even stranger brain zaps. It wasn't widely advertised at the time by drug reps, but it was a side effect of suddenly stopping the then new SSRI antidepressants. It wasn't a side effect of the older generation of antidepressants, so it wasn't obvious at first what was going on. And the drug reps at the time didn't warn me that this could happen.

The condition is now known as discontinuation syndrome. Other effects of suddenly stopping these antidepressants include feeling like you have the flu, nausea, headaches, dizziness, confusion, irritability, agitation and anxiety. The problem is that you may not recognise that this is what is going on. If you stop your antidepressant drugs as you feel you don't need them anymore and start getting these effects, you may think the depression or anxiety is coming back and immediately restart them. Patients take these drugs for years under the illusion that they still need them to treat their depression.

The *Monthly Index of Medical Specialities* (MIMS – an online medical information resource, the doctors' bible for pharmaceutical information) reports these side effects are rare. Yet I doubt it. If a patient either tries to stop their antidepressant or runs out of them and within a day or two starts feeling anxious, irritable, agitated and has difficulty sleeping, I think most people would interpret this to mean that the depression is coming back, and that they still need the medication. I suspect a lot of their doctors would think the same, too. Maybe the electric shocks would be a giveaway and help the doctor's recognition of the problem, but if the patient didn't have those, the discontinuation effect would go unrecognised.

In a New Zealand study of 180 patients on long-term antidepressants 73.5 per cent had experienced withdrawal symptoms, and almost half of those reported that their withdrawal symptoms had been severe.[35]

Even reducing medication at the rate recommended by the pharmaceutical companies can be too quick and result in discontinuation syndrome. The reduction schedule may have to stretch over many weeks, even months, but can be successful at avoiding these unpleasant symptoms.

The former president of the Royal Australian College of General Practitioners (RACGP, the peak body for general practitioners in Australia), Dr Harry Nespolon said, 'This is one of those areas where patients' effect is so variable that guidelines may in fact be incredibly unhelpful.'

This was said in response to new research that confirms what many GPs have concluded for themselves, namely that withdrawing patients from antidepressants is a lot harder than the clinical guidelines suggest.[36]

Regarding discontinuation syndrome the UK guidelines noted that such symptoms were 'usually mild and self-limiting over about one week'. Similarly, the US guidelines suggested that a patient's withdrawal reactions 'typically resolve without specific treatment over one to two weeks'.

However, in a study released in Addiction Behaviours Journal October 2018, researchers found out that this was not true. Backing up the New Zealand study, the researchers stated that 56 per cent of patients trying to come off antidepressants experienced withdrawal effects and 46 per cent of those patients experiencing these withdrawals described them as severe and lasting several *months*.

Though the textbooks say that antidepressants aren't addictive, discontinuation syndrome seems to fit the bill to me.

'THE CLUTCH PEDAL HAS JUST FALLEN OFF'

When I was a kid, Dad bought a brand-new Ford Cortina Mark 1. It was a totally new design and had just come onto the market. It was his pride and joy. The loose bolts and poor paint in various parts were minor annoyances. Then we went out for a drive when it still had only a handful of miles on the clock. Suddenly a huge gush of steam came up from under the bonnet. Dad pulled over immediately. Dad called my handyman grandfather who quickly diagnosed the problem. The radiator hose had blown off the radiator because the clamp was loose-fitting. He efficiently re-joined it and filled the radiator with water. That was a much bigger annoyance than a few rattles. Not many weeks later, we were driving one night and pulled up at a set of traffic lights. The lights turned green, but we didn't move. There was a loud clunk instead. 'The clutch pedal has just fallen off!' Dad cried out in disbelief. Even my granddad couldn't fix that one. He came and took us home while Dad dealt with the tow truck. That was it for him. It wasn't too long after that that Dad traded the car in. It held so much promise, but that car was a lemon.

I don't think post-marketing surveillance and recalls had been thought of in those days. Of course, we have all kinds of safety systems to prevent this now, haven't we? Except, by its very definition that it happens after the goods have been marketed. For example, in 2018, faulty Takata airbags resulted in 3 million cars being recalled in Australia alone. But this recall took place after some 24 people around the world had died and some 244 had been injured by the faulty airbags exploding.[37] The massive recall didn't help those unfortunate people.

We have a similar situation in the pharmaceutical industry. A system of testing, trials and regulations was put in place after the thalidomide disaster in which pregnant women were prescribed thalidomide for nausea and poor sleep. The drug worked well but had the disastrous side effect of causing severe limb deformities and other physical abnormalities in babies. Some 10,000 children were affected.

Like the car industry, post-marketing surveillance in the pharmaceutical industry will only pick up problems *after* the drug has been released to the market. In my time as a GP I have seen several instances of this.

Capoten (captopril) came on the Australian market in the early 1980s to great fanfare. It was the first of a new class of antihypertensives, the ACE inhibitors. I attended a satellite link up at the launch. It seemed the perfect drug. Much more effective than previous antihypertensives. One doctor in the audience, an early adopter of the drug queried the speaker on a side effect he had noted. Several of his patients had developed a persistent dry cough. The speaker downplayed it saying that it was a rare side effect and not a very significant one. The doctor insisted that it was not rare, and that he had several patients with it. The microphone was taken from him.

When I started using the drug, I too found that the cough was not a rare side effect. It seemed to occur in up to a third of my patients on the drug. The cough was harmless, but quite annoying and persistent. It was easy to overlook the side effect, because most people only developed the cough after the time you would normally see the patient at the one-month mark to check their blood pressure and ask how they had been going with the medication. Often the patient would put up with the irritating cough for months, because they had not connected it to taking the medication. It has been demonstrated that the incidence of the cough is 5–35 per cent.[38] The MIMS, which lists the manufacturer's own prescribing notes still today, over thirty years later, lists the incidence of cough as 0.5–2 per cent.

Renitec (enalapril) came onto the Australian market as a same class rival to Capoten. It was promoted by their reps as being less likely to cause a cough. This was supported by a number of specialists quickly switching their prescribing to the newer drug. Time has shown that the incidence of cough is in fact even worse than Capoten: 7 per cent vs 5.1 per cent in one study.[39] Again, the current MIMS lists the incidence of cough in Renitec as 1.3 per cent.

More serious was the case of the drug Vioxx (rofecoxib), which came on the market around the year 2000 from the then-new class of COX-2 inhibitors, touted as being much safer than older non-steroidal anti-inflammatory drugs because they didn't cause peptic ulcers. That was true, however, the manufacturers stalled for five years on revealing to doctors that it doubled the risk of heart attacks. Vioxx was 'voluntarily withdrawn' from the market after causing up to 140,000 heart attacks in the US alone.[40]

Just in case you think that post-marketing surveillance at least picks up any problems promptly, consider the sobering case of Melleril (thioridazine). It was a golden oldie for many years. It came on the market around 1960 and was widely used for schizophrenia and psychotic episodes. It was used in nursing homes to sedate people who were confused and demented until a study in 2001 showed that it was ineffective in dementia and stated, 'If thioridazine were not currently in widespread clinical use, there would be inadequate evidence to support its introduction'.[41] In 2005, *45 years* after its introduction, it was withdrawn worldwide as it was found to cause severe cardiac arrhythmias.

WHO lists 462 medications that have been withdrawn due to post-marketing surveillance detecting serious side effects in the period 1953–2013.[42] That's an average of over seven drugs a year for that 60-year period. WHO also worryingly stated it took on average six years for a drug to be withdrawn. That's six years in which patients are consuming the drug and at risk of a major side effect. They point out also that unfortunately, over that 60-year period, regulatory authorities haven't gotten any quicker at responding to reports of side effects.

There is a principle drummed into doctors in medical school: *primum non nocere*, first do no harm. Over the years I have certainly become less ready to listen to the hype surrounding the release of a new drug. I like to see a proven, clear advantage in a new drug compared to an existing drug before switching. Newer is not necessarily better. By the way, did you know that for a new drug to be approved for use in Australia, the pharmaceutical company is not required to demonstrate that it is any more effective than existing drugs for any particular condition? Perhaps the guiding principle should be changed to *caveat emptor*, let the buyer beware'.

EFFECTS AND SIDE EFFECTS

There is a fine line sometimes between an effect and a side effect. If it is a good result it is called an effect, and if it is a bad result it is called a side effect. Take Zyban (bupropion) for example. It came on the market in the USA around the early 1990s as an antidepressant. It is a norepinephrine and dopamine reuptake inhibitor (NDRI). After a while it was observed that a lot of patients on it unexpectedly experienced a side effect of ceasing cigarette smoking tobacco. The effect was to help relieve depression; the side effect was stopping smoking.

Some ten years later, around 2001, Zyban (bupropion) came on the Australian market and was promoted as a medication to assist in quitting smoking tobacco. Being the first drug to be made available for this, it was avidly used by Australian doctors. Initially, the drug company did not make Australian doctors aware that it had been already in use in the USA for the previous ten years as an antidepressant. The result was that a number of Australian patients already on antidepressants were prescribed Zyban to take as well as their antidepressant, commonly SSRIs or SNRIs. The ensuing interaction between the two drugs could cause agitation, aggressiveness, restlessness and even seizures. So, in Australia, the effect was to stop smoking. Whereas the antidepressant effect was an unwanted side effect.

Because antidepressants inhibit the reuptake of serotonin, norepinephrine or dopamine, the side effects of SSRIs, SNRIs and NDRIs are predictably the effect of excessive serotonin, norepinephrine or dopamine at the receptor sites.

As these receptors are in the brain, that is where most of the side effects are found. Some antidepressants cause drowsiness. If you give that to a depressed person who is already lethargic and tired, the result is a side effect of making them feel even worse. Give it to a depressed person who is agitated, and it slows them down. Then it is promoted as an effect.

Similarly, if you prescribe an antidepressant that tends to hype people up to an agitated depressed person, then this is a side effect as they will feel worse. Give it to a depressed person who is lethargic, and it speeds them up. Then it is promoted as an effect.

The trick is knowing which antidepressant to give to which patient. And the answer is not always straight forward. If you feel that the antidepressant you are taking is causing excessive sedation or agitation, then please discuss this with your doctor.

Other central nervous system side effects include sleep disturbance, weird dreams and dizziness. Blurred vision and or dry eyes are further potential side effects.

Because the various receptors are found throughout the gastrointestinal tract, antidepressants commonly affect this part of the body. So, side effects include dry mouth, nausea, constipation, diarrhoea and weight gain (through increased appetite).

The other part of the body that may be affected is the reproductive system, causing erectile dysfunction and or the inability to orgasm. This could obviously make a bad situation worse, given that people with depression often have a decreased sex drive to start with.

Again, if you believe you may be having (unwanted) side effects from your medication, please discuss this with your doctor. The doctor won't know you are experiencing these if you don't speak up.

THE ULTIMATE DANGER

I think doctors underestimate the powerful effect on the patient of prescribing a drug, whatever the medical problem. It immediately signals to the patient that the doctor has heard them and acknowledged that the patient has a problem that they are taken seriously. Sometimes you can see the relief on patients' faces. It raises hope in the patient that there will soon be an end to their suffering. It also tends to unburden them of the load they are carrying. I think these all invoke the placebo response.

Although this may make them feel better in the short term, I believe that it can be disempowering for the patient. The problem can be that patients see their depression as the doctor's problem to fix and not their problem any longer. There is a disincentive for them to sort through the issues that triggered the depression in the first place.

And I think doctors and medical authorities are complicit in this. Depression of all degrees, mild as well as moderate and severe, is seen as a medical problem, and like all medical problems, it requires a medical solution.

5

WHAT CROHN'S DISEASE TAUGHT ME ABOUT THE MODERN MEDICAL MODEL

In 1979 I graduated in medicine with honours from what I considered the best university in Australia, the University of Sydney. I had accepted what I had learned from my professors and began practising conventional medicine. Not that I thought of it as conventional. It was medicine that I practised, based on clear understanding of how the body worked. I knew of no other.

I commenced general practice in Coffs Harbour, a seaside town halfway between Sydney and Brisbane, in 1982. I practised with the certainty of youth, until I reached a personal health crisis ten years later. I developed Crohn's disease, which caused me severe abdominal pain. When I say severe, I mean the first episode of abdominal pain came on so suddenly and severely that I had to pull my car over to the curb and I fell out onto the ground on all fours. I broke out in a profuse cold sweat. The vice-like gripping pain increased in intensity until I was praying for God to take my life immediately. The level of pain had gone from 0 out of 10 to 10 out of 10 in the space of a couple of minutes. I lost 6kg in the following week, yet I took only one day off work. I continued to ignore my symptoms for the next two years in my workaholic state until I literally collapsed at work one day. The Crohn's disease had caused a fistula (a hole in the wall of the intestine) and two abscesses, each 10 cm (four inches) in diameter. After a week of intravenous antibiotics I underwent major surgery with the removal of 60cm (24 inches) of small intestine and the ascending colon. It came as a complete shock to me that this was necessary. I saw no connection between my workaholic lifestyle and my illness.

Prior to my illness, my practice of medicine had become finely honed and I had gotten faster and faster at assessing and managing medical problems. The consultations became shorter and shorter, and my workdays became longer and longer. I hadn't taken a holiday for four years. At that time, I did not have an appointment system and it would not be unusual to have ten or more patients sitting in the waiting room to see me, and I didn't like to keep people waiting. I was trying to meet an insatiable demand, seeing over 250 patients per week. The week I collapsed had seemed like a victory, as I had seen 299 patients that week. It was very easy to diagnose tonsillitis and prescribe penicillin. Next! A chest infection, Amoxil and a cough expectorant. Next! Gastroenteritis, a light diet and Imodium. Next! Depressed? An antidepressant. What's wrong with this picture?

Following my surgery, I asked the surgeon if I should go on any special diet or take vitamins, especially as I had lost over 20kg in weight. (I was so thin at the time, many of my patients told me that they thought I had cancer.) The surgeon said that I could eat anything I wanted and didn't need to take any vitamins because I was cured. My surgeon was highly skilled. I have no doubt about that. But that doesn't mean he was highly skilled in everything – just what he was trained for, to operate. Within six weeks my symptoms of abdominal pain started to return.

A friend of mine, a medical doctor and member of the Australasian College of Nutritional and Environmental Medicine (ACNEM), suggested the then unusual treatment of megadoses of vitamins and minerals, together with radical changes to my diet, including the elimination of dairy, gluten, sugar and nuts. Despite the rather restrictive diet I gained weight and felt a whole lot more energetic. And the pain went away.

After these amazing results, the main question that went through my mind was, 'Why wasn't I taught about this in medical school?' I thought that I had been taught a complete understanding of the body. I now felt that I had been cheated. I began to see that medicine is brilliant at managing acute and life-threatening situations, but it is rather poor at managing chronic disease. The focus is on the pathogen or disease process, to the virtual exclusion of the condition of the body itself, let alone that body's mind or spirit.

Thus began my journey of discovery in complementary therapies. I attended the primary course for ACNEM and my eyes were opened to a huge range of possibilities that had never been discussed in medical school.

However, the following year, I had a further recurrence of the Crohn's disease, and was required to go onto three months of high-dose steroids. I had seen what high-dose steroids had done to numerous patients of mine, so this propelled me to search even more deeply into alternatives. I began seeing a number of health professionals skilled in various complementary health modalities and attended an inner-child workshop, learned counselling and communication skills, acupuncture and cognitive behaviour therapy.

I realised that various traditions and techniques allow us to see human beings from a different perspective. Each discipline has its own language to describe what is going on within us. Each discipline has its own strengths and its own weaknesses. None of these disciplines, including conventional Western medicine, can describe the totality of what is going on within each one of us.

I am reminded of the body maps described by the Ancient One in the film *Doctor Strange*. The Ancient One showed Dr Strange three maps of the body: the chakras, the acupuncture meridians and an MRI, and told him, 'Each of those maps was drawn up by someone who could see in part but not the whole. You are a man who has been looking through a keyhole and has spent his whole life trying to widen the keyhole to see more, to know more.'

By the late 1990s I came to a realisation in the core of my being that I had developed Crohn's disease because deep down I had thought of myself as gutless. It was a painful lesson, but I finally came to learn to trust my gut instincts. It is hard to explain the difference between knowing at an intellectual level and knowing in the core of my being. That 'knowing' resulted in a huge shift for me in mind, body and spirit. I have been on a journey ever since that major life crisis a quarter of a century ago, driven by an insatiable curiosity to understand what the human body is and how it works.

Transformational Acupuncture is one modality that focuses the mind to have realisations – ah-ha moments. From my personal experience, the new thought (about how a situation is viewed) is always accompanied by a strong emotional reaction or release. It can be a flood of love and compassion flowing from the heart, the release of bottled-up grief associated with a release of tears, or the release of anger and frustration (often aimed at a significant other or family of origin), but it is then followed by a sense of inner peace.

By the way, I have not had a recurrence of Crohn's since 1994. Interestingly, in all the years that I've had follow-up checks with specialists, not one has ever asked me about my diet or supplements or having acupuncture. Oh, except one specialist, who years ago asked, 'Are you still taking all that funny stuff?'

6

BODY MAPS – WHERE
EAST MEETS WEST

Like Dr Stephen Strange the Marvel character, most medically trained people in the West are brought up, as I was, with the biomedical model of looking at the body. It doesn't occur to most that there are other ways of looking at the complexity of human beings.

THE WESTERN BIOMEDICAL MODEL

The biomedical model has been around for nearly two centuries. What is the biomedical model? This views a healthy human being as one who is free of disease, defects and pain. And if you are not free of disease, defects and pain, there is something wrong with you. You go to a doctor to find out what is wrong. The doctor takes a history, performs an examination and may order a number of investigations to come to a conclusion of what is 'wrong' with you: the diagnosis. Doctors then prescribe medicines to alleviate or correct what is wrong. If they can't 'fix it' with medications, you are then referred to a surgeon to cut out, repair or replace the defective part.

In a large percentage of cases this works and works well. I can recall, with great satisfaction, giving one particular patient a course of penicillin and seeing them recover from life-threatening pneumonia. Or another patient who had a shattered ear from being thrown through a car window. I spent an hour or two in emergency department one night figuring out how to put the ear back together with 49 sutures. Then being complimented the next day by the plastic-surgery team on my handiwork. Or the time an unconscious truck driver was brought in by ambulance with his right arm hanging on by a thread. He had a compound fracture of his humerus. The only thing holding his arm together was the neurovascular bundle, basically a string of gristle. Amazingly, his wrist had a pulse. I assisted the surgeon to put it back together. A couple of weeks later the truck driver left hospital a happy man with a fully functioning right arm. It gave me an incredible buzz to feel that I made a difference in someone's life.

Sometimes the process is straight forward like in these cases, sometimes not so straight forward. Sometimes the process seems to fail. I have lost count how many times over the years I have seen a patient with symptoms of chronic fatigue syndrome, and they tell me with disgust that their previous doctor told them, despite their debilitating symptoms, 'There's nothing wrong with you.' This happens when the doctor relies on the investigations alone. If they show no abnormality, their conclusion is that there is no sign of disease or defect and conclude that 'there is nothing wrong'. This assumes that investigations can tell you everything there is to know about the patient. This is patently false. Let's conduct a thought experiment. Twin brothers present for examination. The day before one of them ran a marathon in a personal best, while the other sat on the couch and enjoyed watching a game of footy. Which brother ran the marathon? The doctor is allowed to perform any examination and order any investigation to make a determination. The truth is there is no test available that will show a difference. Yet the brother who ran the marathon will certainly feel different from the one who didn't. The fact that all the tests

THE WESTERN BIOMEDICAL MODEL

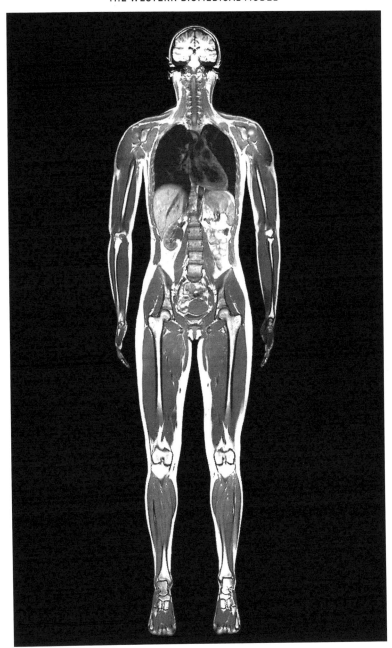

would be negative doesn't mean that the runner wouldn't feel exhausted and achy, that it is 'all in his head'. We can use a battery meter and determine the amount of charge in an AA battery, but we can't measure the amount of energy in a human body.

What if the doctor saw a patient with chronic fatigue who said they could barely get out of bed or do a few chores and yet felt totally exhausted? What then? If the focus is on the pain, increasingly strong analgesics are prescribed until the patient is eventually put on chronic opioids. If the patient breaks down and cries about their symptoms often enough (especially a female patient with a male doctor), they will end up on antidepressants.

With the biomedical model of the body, the doctor views the human body as a mechanic views a car. They both see a machine with functioning parts and broken parts. The doctor just focuses on the specific body part concerned and treats it as car mechanic would investigate an unusual noise coming from under the hood. But humans aren't cars, we are vastly more complex – and self-repairing to boot. There are other ways of viewing the body than this mechanistic method.

THE TRADITIONAL CHINESE MODEL

The traditional Chinese model of the human body seems to be completely contradictory and irrelevant to the modern scientific mind. Yet it has stood the test of time, being used to treat a variety of ailments over the past two thousand years or more. The *Ling Shu*, or *Divine Pivot*, is the first known book on acupuncture. The concept of pivot is that you can bring about great change from a point: i.e. have an influence on an organ or even the whole body from a point, the acupuncture point. The text is dated around the first century BCE and presents acupuncture virtually as it is today. This suggests that the origin of acupuncture is much earlier than

THE TRADITIONAL CHINESE MODEL

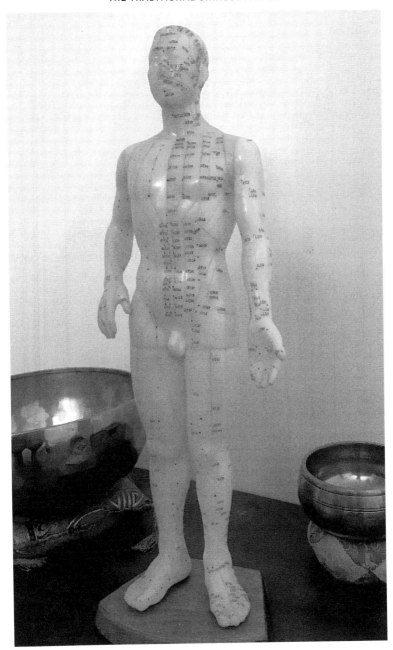

that. (The text is still in use today and I get a kick out of having a translation of this ancient text on my twenty-first-century Kindle.)

When I first heard lectures on acupuncture, it didn't make sense to my medically trained mind. I often argued with myself about what I was hearing. What does the spleen have to do with sugar? If the patient had spleen Qi deficiency, why did that cause dampness in the body, i.e. fluid retention? It took me quite a while to make sense of what it was all about. It is important to realise that the ancient Chinese had a rudimentary understanding of the anatomy of the body. This was due largely to the fact that it was against their beliefs to perform post-mortems.

But it's not just a different view of anatomy that results in such a different view of the body. The traditional Chinese model is based on a different philosophy. The West and the East have quite different views of the world, let alone the human form. These views diverged over two millennia ago.

Western philosophy is largely based on that of ancient Greece. In particular, the logical reasoning of Aristotle (c. 384–322 BCE) has resulted in the concept of contraries, two propositions where both cannot be true: my cat is black; my cat is white. Logically, both statements cannot be true. Doctors use this concept in medicine all the time. For example, the gall bladder is diseased; the gall bladder is not diseased. Logically, both statements cannot be true. If a patient presents with right upper quadrant pain, doctors begin with history and examination, then imaging to determine the truth. Histology is the final arbiter, when the surgeon sends the gall bladder to the pathology laboratory following surgery. Generally, this serves us well. In keeping with the biomedical model, we classify someone as having a disease or not.

However, does the patient have hypertension or not? Does the patient have diabetes or not? Does the patient have hypercholesterolaemia (high cholesterol) or not? There really is no clear-cut division between patient with these conditions or not. When I graduated, the cut-off for hypercholesterolaemia was a cholesterol reading over 6.5 mmol/l. Anything below that was considered normal, while above was pathological. That cut-off point was reduced to 6.0, then 5.5, then 5.4 and now stands at 5.2. Clearly, the pathological process of cholesterol in human beings has not changed over the years. This is an arbitrary cut-off point based on statistics of a whole population.

The concept is that patients with readings above a predetermined level should be treated, while those below should not. Doctors are trying to separate the population into 'the diseased' and 'the not diseased'. The reality is that a percentage of people will be treated unnecessarily, and some people who ultimately should be treated aren't. Doctors can only quote the statistics, the number needed to treat to prevent a certain outcome like a heart attack or stroke.

For example, by giving whole populations cholesterol-lowering statins we can prevent one in 217 from having a non-fatal heart attack and one in 313 from having a non-fatal stroke. That may sound good if we can prevent these conditions, but that means 200–300 people will be taking that medication unnecessarily for every one person who is helped, and at great cost to health as well as monetarily. For one in 21 will experience pain from muscle damage, and one in 204 will develop diabetes mellitus as side effect of taking the medication. At the same time, *no* fatal heart attacks or strokes are prevented.[43] (Please note, the statistics are quite different for secondary prevention in those who already have had a heart attack or stroke, where statins have proven their worth.)

The biomedical model of disease or not diseased does not work well in this situation. We have similar circumstances with blood pressure readings in diagnosing hypertension and with glucose readings in diagnosing diabetes. We are talking about a couple of billion people with these three conditions alone. What is the solution?

Rather than seeing things in black or white, the Chinese focused their attention for more than two millennia on understanding the body in terms of a healthy balanced function compared with a pathological excessive or deficient function. This comes directly from the Chinese concept of Yin–Yang as a philosophical means of describing the universe and everything in it, including the human body.

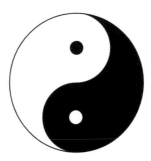

This famous symbol summarises the concept of Yin and Yang contained within the whole. Yin is representative of cool, while Yang is warmth; Yin is female, Yang is male; Yin is quiet, stillness, nurturing and building up, anabolic, while Yang is loud, energetic, action, catabolic. And so forth.

At first glance the Yin and the Yang are seen by Westerners as the familiar opposites of black or white, but the Chinese see much more. Together Yin and Yang form the whole, a unity, signified by being contained within a circle. Nothing is all Yin or all Yang. Imbalance will cause illness. If you are on the go all the time, too much Yang, you will become exhausted. If you stay in bed for many days, your muscles will waste away. The ideal is a balance between activity and rest. This balance isn't static, but constantly changing. The wavy line down the middle signifies this constant state of flux. Nothing is static in the body. They are complementary. One cannot exist without the other. The line is wavy not an impenetrable straight wall dividing the circle in half.

There is always a kernel of Yin within Yang, and Yang within Yin, which can result in sudden change from one to another. A simple example of this is the sudden feeling of chills when one starts out with a high fever. This is symbolised by the small dot of opposite colour within each part in the diagram.

The Chinese anticipated the discovery of the autonomic nervous system and the concept of homeostasis by some two thousand years. For more information on this see my book *Stick it to Depression: Another Tool in Your Doctor's Bag.*

Over time, as I learned some of the basics of Chinese medicine, I found myself looking at a patient from a Western medical approach and coming up with a diagnosis, then looking at the same patient from a Chinese medical approach and coming up with a diagnosis in that system. Sometimes I found the Chinese diagnosis more helpful from a management point of view, especially when the diagnosis wasn't clear from a Western medical point of view.

I was reminded of this when a patient presented to me some years ago with a diagnosis of sciatica. He had seen the neurosurgeon and was on his waiting list to have a back operation. The patient came to me hoping that acupuncture would at least give some pain relief in the meantime. After examining the patient, I agreed with the neurosurgeon's diagnosis. Yet from the Chinese perspective it seemed to me like the patient had a blockage in the gall bladder channel, that runs down the lateral aspect of the leg. According to Chinese theory, that channel is internally connected to the gall bladder and I agree that doesn't make any sense from a Western viewpoint. And what exactly is blocked? Yet when I needled the appropriate acupuncture points to unblock the channel, the patient got some relief of pain. Over the next few weeks, the patient fully recovered and cancelled his planned surgery! I suggested to the patient that cutting his fat and alcohol intake and reducing his weight might prevent a recurrence.

It is those occasions that give me an appreciation that my understanding of the Chinese theory of acupuncture can give me a different view of the same human body in Western medicine. And sometimes that view can offer insights not seen by Western medicine. And it has also driven me to suggest a trial of acupuncture to patients first before something as drastic as surgery.

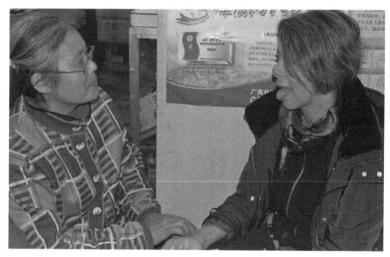

A 'barefoot doctor' in a village near Guilin observes the tongue and feels the pulse in 2012.

THE INDIAN AYURVEDIC MODEL

You may look at this map of the body and think, 'OK you have had me following you so far, but now you've lost me. How does this 'map' of the body even relate to the real world let alone to medicine?'

THE INDIAN AYURVEDIC MODEL

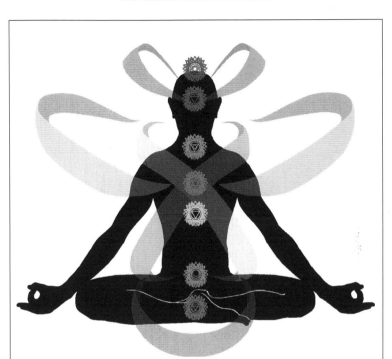

The Indian Ayurvedic Model showing the seven chakras or energy centres, from the 1st at the base of the spine to the 7th at the crown of the head. Drawn by Peter Lagettie

In the Indian Ayurvedic model, there are seven chakras. On one level these can be seen as spiritual power centres, as suggested by the Indian mystics, or as energy centres that are associated with the central nervous system. These concepts have evolved over time, particularly over the last hundred years. Westerners have associated the chakras with the various nerve plexuses and centres, and also with the various endocrine organs. More than one person has seen the similarity in the spiritual qualities of the chakras (from safety/survival of the root chakra, through to enlightenment of the crown chakra) and Maslow's hierarchy of needs as a way of understanding human motivation.

For details, see *Rainbow Body: A History of the Western Chakra System from Blavatsky to Brennan* by Kurt Leland.

What is the value in considering the Ayurvedic body map? I see the value in attempting to link the body to the mind and the spirit. In the following table I have attempted to draw parallels between the modern medical model, the traditional Chinese model and the Indian Ayurvedic model.

We generally don't think much about the autonomic nervous system in general practice, but the various ganglia and plexuses of nerves act as mini-brains co-ordinating the myriad of autonomic functions in the body. This allows us not to consciously have to think of what blood pressure changes we need to control throughout our arterial tree when we stand up, when we lie down, when we go for a run. We don't have to be concerned about when and how much stomach juices we produce when we eat a meal, or when to contract the gall bladder to release the detergents to break up the fat in our half-digested meal. We don't need to raise a sweat thinking about how much perspiration we need to produce to maintain our core temperature at any given moment. We don't need to consciously open up our irises when we walk down a dark lane.

I say 'mini-brains' because although most of their functions are continuously happening in the background at an unconscious level, sometimes their functioning rises to the level just below or at the level of consciousness.

These basic autonomic functions are going on 24/7, but our central nervous system is even more amazingly built than that, and even higher functions can happen automatically. I remember when I took my first driving lessons back in the 1970s. It was overwhelming to think, 'OK, I've checked for cars in the rear mirror.

CORRELATION BETWEEN THE THREE DIFFERENT MODELS

Chakra No.	Sanskrit Name	Translation	Western Name	Nerve Centre	Endocrine Organ	Spiritual Qualities	Maslow's Hierarchy of Needs	Location Anteriorly	Location Posteriorly
								Traditional Chinese Acupoints	
7	Sahasrara	Thousand Petaled	Crown	Frontal Lobe	Pineal Gland	Enlightenment	Self-Transcendence	GV20	GV20
6	Ajna	Command	Third Eye	Hypothalamus	Pituitary Gland	Intuition Imagination	Self-Actualisation	Yintang	GV16
5	Vishuddha	Especially Pure	Throat	Laryngeal/ Pharyngeal	Thyroid/ Parathyroid Glands	Communication Creative Expression	Self-Actualisation	CV22	GV14
4	Anahata	Unstruck Unhurt Unbeaten	Heart	Cardiac Plexus	Heart	Unconditional Love	Esteem	CV17	GV11
3	Manipura	Lustrous Gem	Solar Plexus	Solar Plexus	Pancreas	Personal Power Relationship to others	Esteem	CV10	GV8
2	Svadhishthana	Where your being is established	Sacral or Sex	Prostatic/ Vaginal Plexus	Gonads	Sexuality Relationship with partner	Love/Belonging	CV4	GV4
1	Muladhara	Root and basis of existence	Root	Sacral	Adrenals/ Kidneys	Survival Grounding Relationship with oneself	Safety/ Physiological	GV1	GV1

I've got my right foot on the brake and my left on the clutch. I've got my indicator on. The gear stick is in first gear.' Then totally focus on easing the left foot off the clutch until it engaged. I'd be feeling pretty good about remembering all of that then, embarrassingly, start kangaroo hopping down the road. Before you know it, I'd have to think about changing from first to second gear. I think you would agree those first few hours of driving were pretty stressful. Imagine if every time you drove your car since it was like those first few hours? How would you listen to music or a podcast while driving? How would you have time to think about all the things you needed to do when you got to your office? Let alone observing what the traffic was doing around you, or checking the traffic lights, and speedometer, all while having a deep and meaningful conversation with your passenger. Have you ever driven across town while deep in thought and suddenly realised that you had driven several kilometres and not remembered any of the journey? And yet you had, obviously, successfully navigated all those streets, intersections and traffic lights. Fortunately, your mini-brains are working well.

Sometimes one mini-brain dominates. The root chakra that the Ayurvedic places at the base of the spine concerns security and safety. It will swing into action automatically without hesitation when danger strikes. When my older daughter was a young teenager, we went down the paddock to see the newest member of our family, a new-born calf. The mother cow took exception at how close my daughter got to her calf and motioned to chase her. It only took what seemed a couple of seconds for my daughter to race to the nearest tree and climb the first few branches. I had never seen her move so fast before, and haven't since! On a more serious note, decorum goes out the window if in a crowded stadium a fire breaks out. People can behave irrationally and selfishly. Don't try and stand in the way of a panicking crowd. I have often witnessed a distressed and severely anxious person in my clinic. They can literally not be able to sit down but have to pace up and down the room. I think this is an effect of the survival mini-brain being active.

I could go on and on, but one other example of the value of looking at the body from the three different body maps, is that of the heart.

We generally think of the heart as merely a pump. It may be a sophisticated, but a pump nonetheless. If functioning is impaired, it may beat irregularly, or it may beat weakly in heart failure, particularly if its own blood supply is impaired. But there are two other aspects of the heart that are generally ignored.

Firstly, the heart is an endocrine organ. This fact was first recognised in 1984 with the discovery of atrial natriuretic peptide (ANP).[44]

Since then the heart has been demonstrated to produce brain natriuretic peptide (BNP), C-type natriuretic peptide, adrenomedullin, proadrenomedullin N-terminal peptide and endothelin-1.[45]

More recently, the heart has also been shown to produce a couple of dozen hormones, including the catecholamines: adrenalin (epinephrine), noradrenalin (norepinephrine) and dopamine.[46]

Importantly, the heart has been shown to produce oxytocin.[47] Oxytocin has been called 'the love hormone' as blood levels have been shown to rise in sexual activity, childbirth and breast feeding, as well as even hugging.

Also important is that the heart has been shown to produce serotonin.[48] Low levels of serotonin in the brain is, of course, implicated in depression. The Heart Foundation released a document in 2012 (see following page) warning that 'people with depression could be at greater risk of heart disease'. Traditional Chinese medicine has understood this link for the last two thousand years. Traditional Chinese medicine has associated heart problems with a lack of joy in life. Modern medicine is just catching up.

2012 MEDIA RELEASE FROM THE HEART FOUNDATION

Media Release

5 January 2012

Australian research on heart disease and depression

People with depression could be at greater risk of heart disease, according to an international research team led by a Charles Sturt University researcher.

Dr Robert Grenfell, National Clinical Issues Director at the National Heart Foundation of Australia, said the study confirmed the importance of treating depression to avoid heart disease.

"We know that depression, social isolation and lack of quality support is a key risk factor for cardiovascular disease and this study confirms the importance of us treating it in its early stages," he said.

More than 46,000 Australians die each year from cardiovascular disease, Australia's number one killer.

The study found that depression seemed to change the way heart rate is controlled, which increases the risk of heart attack. The authors also found that diabetes seemed to worsen the risk of cardiac arrest in people with depression.

"Mild depression is associated with doubling the risk of developing cardiovascular disease and heart attack (and death from these causes), and severe depression has an even more profound effect - with up to five times the rate of cardiovascular disease as compared to non-depressed people," Dr Grenfell said.

"Unfortunately, evidence from large studies where depression appears to be adequately treated, have not shown any reversal, or improvement in the cardiovascular disease risk

"Therefore the best option is to treat depression in its early stages," he said.

Those suffering from depression are reminded that it can be treated with medical and non-medical therapies. The Heart Foundation encourages anyone concerned about depression to call their health professional as a first step.

More information on the risk factors for cardiovascular disease is available at the Heart Foundation website. http://www.heartfoundation.org.au/your-heart/know-the-risks/Pages/default.aspx

Interestingly, three randomised controlled trials have looked to see if treating depression lessens the risk of heart disease:

- in 2003 ENRICHD – enhancing recovery in coronary heart disease using CBT and group therapy;
- in 2005 SADHART – CHF – sertraline against depression and heart disease in chronic heart failure; and
- in 2007 CREATE – Canadian cardiac randomised evaluation of antidepressant (citalopram) and psychotherapy efficacy.

All three resulted in an improvement in symptoms, but all three failed to reduce the incidence of heart symptoms. Perhaps it is because they are looking at the heart problem as being secondary to the depressive disorder rather than the other way around – or at least both having a common underlying cause. That is to say the SSRIs or counselling are mere band-aids and doesn't get to the root of the problem of why patients lack joy in their lives.

Besides understanding the importance of the heart as a fully-fledged endocrine gland, the heart has a plexus of nerves at the base, the cardiac plexus. Western doctors think of the vagus nerve sending para-sympathetic signals to slow the heart rate. But the vagus nerve carries more afferent (sensory) signals back to the brain than efferent (motor) signals to the heart. We really do experience heart-felt feelings. Anyone who has fallen in love will vouch for that. Unless they are cold-hearted or have a heart of stone!

One of my first experiences of acupuncture was a few months after my first wife died of breast cancer. The acupuncture points used on me were heart points. During the session, my thoughts turned to her and after a while I experienced what I could only describe as angina. It felt like a heaviness in my chest, radiating up into my throat as a tightness and accompanied by some tears in my eyes. It lasted only about 30 seconds or so, and was immediately followed by a few skipped beats, then a lightness in my chest. I felt a sensation of letting her go. This was followed by a strong sense of calm and peace.

I have had patients describe similar events to me after their treatments. I think this results in real healing. I would love to do a study on this. I currently have an octogenarian female patient, Janelle, who I had been treating with acupuncture for post-herpetic neuralgia, a chronic unrelenting pain after an attack of shingles. She had great relief of symptoms with that. Later, after her partner of many years died, she developed depression. After some months, she recalled that the acupuncture had made her generally feel well, so she returned for acupuncture to help her symptoms of depression. Janelle has been attending regularly and reports that she not only no longer feels depressed, she also hardly gets angina anymore. She rarely needs the nitro spray. I'm not saying her heart is normal. She is still on the appropriate treatment for atrial fibrillation and nitro-patches for the angina as well has having a pacemaker, but her cardiologist is happy that her heart is functioning well. She has been quite stable for a few years. She incidentally mentioned to me recently that she doesn't experience panic attacks (which the Chinese relate to heart imbalance) anymore. Although I have been her GP for more than 30 years, she had been too embarrassed to mention them to me.

So we see in this patient the three aspects of the heart: as a mechanical pump; as a bundle of nerves, a nerve plexus, and as an endocrine organ. This is a much more complete picture of the heart.

Likewise, the vagus nerve is carrying afferent (sensory) signals from the other abdominal organs as well. Having a gut-feeling or butterflies in the stomach are real sensations. Too much of our education is based on left-brain thinking; at least it was for me. I was taught to ignore my feelings, to my detriment, as I explained in the chapter about having Crohn's disease.

We don't have any problem understanding that the big toe will let you know immediately if you have stubbed it. But a lot of us have a hard time believing that our heart will tell us if a situation doesn't feel right. It just doesn't seem logical for a mere pump to be speaking to us. Modern medicine is still stuck in the nineteenth-century world of chemistry. It fails to acknowledge the revolution that occurred in physics, now over one hundred years ago with the post-Newtonian world of Einstein. The heart generates electric signals some sixty times stronger than the brain, as measured by an ECG compared with an EEG. Sensitive equipment can measure the heart's magnetic field some feet away. It is 100 times stronger than the brain's magnetic field. Studies have demonstrated the interaction of people's hearts' magnetic fields interacting with one another.[49] We really can have a heart-to-heart conversation. The electromagnetic field of a calm parent's heart really can slow down the heart of an upset infant.

WHAT'S DESCARTES GOT TO DO WITH IT?

Since the time of the French philosopher René Descartes, 1596–1650, Western scientists have separated mind, body and spirit. The focus in medical science has definitely been on the body, with the mind coming a poor second. Psychiatry is still seen as a bit of a Cinderella speciality ("A UK term of dubious utility for any under-appreciated, under-funded or under-discussed specialty" – Medical-Dictionaryt.thefreedictionary.com[50]) in medicine. Meanwhile, the spirit has traditionally been the territory of the Church and has been ignored by medical science. This aspect has withered throughout the twentieth century and has declined even further in the first two decades of the twenty-first century.

Even in 2020 the emotional, spiritual and psychological aspects of human health continue to be ignored by health authorities fixated on the biomedical model. For example, UK doctors are encouraged to 'improve the quality of care their patients are given by rewarding practices for the quality of care they provide to their patients' by setting targets via the Quality and Outcomes Framework (QOF).

Of the 559 indicators measured, only ten indicators relate to depression, the number-one health problem in the world. These points are awarded if a newly diagnosed depressed patient is merely followed up by the GP recording a consultation 10–56 days after diagnosis.[51]

By comparison, diabetes mellitus has 86 indicators, relating to measuring blood pressure, cholesterol, HbA1c (a measure of diabetic control), percentage of diabetics on certain medications, examination of the feet for diabetic damage etc. These are all concrete and easily measured, compared with measuring happiness and fulfillment.

As long as we only think in terms of biochemistry and pathology, we will not have an understanding of some of the mysteries in life. And I don't think we will have an understanding of such a healing modality as acupuncture. I think that being able to view the body from the different aspects of the three traditions of Western medicine, Chinese medicine and Indian Ayurvedic medicine helps to broaden our thinking and opens up the possibilities for healing that we need to explore.

7

WHAT IS A DASS?

Before looking at case studies, I think it appropriate to explain what a DASS is. DASS is an acronym for Depression Anxiety Stress Scale. As you can see from the questionnaire on the following page, it is a list of questions that relate to how depressed, anxious and/or stressed a person is.

The person answers each question based on how they have felt over the previous week. The long version, the DASS42, has 42 questions, and the shortened form, the DASS21, which I use as it is quicker for a person to complete, has 21 questions.

Within the 21 questions there are seven questions relating to depression, seven questions relating to anxiety and seven questions relating to stress. The three types of question are jumbled up to try to avoid the 'donkey vote'. Given that each question has a maximum score of three, that means levels of depression, anxiety and stress are each rated out of a maximum score of 21. This has been validated as a tool both in the research setting as well as the clinical setting, in a large number of countries and in a variety of languages, including Chinese, Turkish, Albanian, to name a few, as well as across the English-speaking world.

The DASS21 can usually be completed in less than five minutes. So, this a quick way to see how a patient has been emotionally over the previous week. Try it for yourself (www.scu.edu.au/media/ scueduau/current-students/services/counselling/downloads/ Depression-Anxiety-Stress-Scales-DASS3481.pdf or onlineclinic. blackdoginstitute.org.au/). Don't think too long about each question. Usually your first thought is correct. Answer each question by circling 0, 1, 2 or 3:

0 if you haven't had that problem
1 if that problem has been mild or infrequent
2 if that problem has been moderate or reasonably regularly
3 if that problem has been severe or constant over the whole week.

When you have finished answering the 21 questions, write the number you have circled for each answer in the corresponding white box to the right of each question. When you have done that for each of the 21 questions, then add up the numbers for each of the three columns D, A and S and write them in the three boxes next to totals at the bottom right.

	Depression	Anxiety	Stress
Normal	0–4	0–3	0–7
Mild	5–6	4–5	8–9
Moderate	7–10	6–7	10–12
Severe	11–13	8–9	13–16
Extremely severe	14+	10+	17+

Please note firstly that this is *not* a diagnostic tool; that is, one can't diagnose major depressive disorder, anxiety disorder and so forth from this tool. But it is an excellent guide as to the severity of symptoms and to monitor progress.

Secondly, it is important to note that this is not even a fixed categorisation of severity. The numbers can bounce around from week to week depending on what is happening in your life and how you interpret them. What seems like a total catastrophe one day may be viewed as a blessing by you another day.

Thirdly, and most importantly, if you find yourself scoring highly, please don't ignore this. Discuss these results with your medical practitioner or psychologist for further advice.

I use this tool, as do a large number of doctors around the world, to give some objectivity to monitoring the progress of a patient. In the following case studies, I have graphed the DASS scores of those patients as a guide to their progress.

8

CASE STUDIES

With my wife's urging to prove that the Transformational Acupuncture treatments were helping depression, I followed five of my patients with depression over a period of a year:

CASE 1:
FIRST EPISODE OF DEPRESSION, FOLLOWING HEAD INJURY

A 45-year-old female shop owner who had a horse-riding accident about 18 months prior to coming to me

She was thrown from her horse and hit her head causing a subdural haematoma and multiple orbital fractures. She'd required two decompressive operations that week and four months later had a cranioplasty. Physically, she seemed to recover, including her memory, but she totally had lost confidence and was unable to work. She felt anxious and often woke up during the night with panic attacks. She felt stressed, which was compounded by the fact that she was no longer able to monetarily support her artist husband. After a year of ongoing symptoms of depression, anxiety and stress, she went to her GP who started her on Efexor XR 75mg (venlafaxine). She felt no significant relief, though her friends told her she seemed to improve as far as they were concerned. She also saw a psychologist but didn't feel any benefit from that. Further assessment confirmed a diagnosis of non-melancholic depression. Non-melancholic depression, which accounts for about 90 per cent of cases of depression, relates to the fact that external factors have triggered the depression in a person who has previously been generally mentally well, but then find themselves not coping with a life stressor. In this case, the stressor was the riding accident, with the resultant head injury.

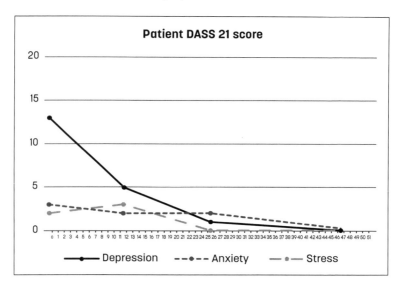

The graph here shows her DASS scores as related by time in weeks from me initially seeing her. The solid line represents the depression. As I said before, each of these scores are out of a maximum of 21. Her score for depression was initially 13. As you can tell from the table in the previous chapter her depression rated as severe. This was a case of pure depression, a feeling of hopelessness, feeling stuck, unable to move forward or see any light on the horizon. As she had been on Efexor for six months prior to this, that would suggest that the medication was not very effective.

As is my usual custom, I gave her a treatment of Transformational Acupuncture at that initial consultation. I find that rather than spending a long time discussing what the acupuncture will do for them, it is better for the patient to actually experience it for themselves. It saves me a lot of talking! Anyway, when I next saw her, she said that when she was driving home after the acupuncture treatment, she found herself singing in the car, which was something she hadn't done for a long, long time. She was thrilled with this. After the second treatment, she said that she had released a lot of anger and she cried like she hadn't cried for years.

After giving her a total of ten sessions, I re-scored her with the DASS21, which showed a reduction in the depression score from 13 to 5, meaning mild depression. She reported that she was living less in the past. She had a further six sessions over the next 16 weeks and the scores had all come down to normal. Around the 20-week mark, which was six weeks prior to that score, she had stopped her antidepressants without my knowledge. She did get one of the side effects with withdrawing from antidepressants, which is electric shock sensations, so-called discontinuation syndrome. Fortunately, the unpleasant sensations faded over a period of one week. She hasn't had any further sessions since the 26th week. So, a total of 16 sessions over 26 weeks. I phoned her around week 47 to see how she was going, and she reported, 'Everything is great. I have so much energy. I'm very happy. It's a miracle.' Her DASS21 score was 0-0-0.

This case illustrates a common scenario. The patient didn't have any real history of depression in the past. She did have some psychological issues with distant parents, distant in a sense of never being warm with her, as well as physical distance – they lived on the other side of the world. She was under constant pressure with being the breadwinner of the house with an artist husband who wasn't bringing in money and having to raise a family, but she generally had found that she coped with these situations over the 24 years of marriage. It wasn't until a major accident that she found that she was unable to cope and became depressed because she didn't see any way out of the situation that she was in. As far as she was concerned, the sessions of acupuncture transformed her life. The antidepressants had only made a mild improvement in her symptoms and she didn't feel like she was going anywhere with them.

She didn't see the relevance of talking with a psychologist about things that had happened in her childhood. It didn't seem relevant to what was happening in her life now. The beauty of acupuncture is that she didn't have to talk about any of this. She figured this all out for herself. I just gave her the acupuncture and her head cleared. Her mood improved, and she got a better perspective on things. She was then able to express emotions, release emotions and feel a sense of optimism and hope that things were getting better. The acupuncture empowered her to solve her own problems or see solutions to her own problems, and helped the negative thoughts swirling around in her mind to disappear.

At 45 years of age, life was beginning to look good to her again. With her new-found clarity of mind, she was able to come up with some solutions with her husband. She got him to help out with working in her shop. She was able to bring up the issue about her not seeing her family for many, many years. The patient and her husband ended up taking a holiday to Europe to meet up with her family again, where she resolved a number of issues with both her parents and her sister.

CASE 2:
EMOTIONALLY OVERWHELMED, WHILE CARRYING THE BURDEN OF A CHRONIC ENERGY-DRAINING PHYSICAL CONDITION

A 47-year-old female, a hard-working dairy farmer and housewife

If you know about dairy farming, you would realise that this is a 24-hour, seven days a week, 52 weeks a year job – including Christmas day. Adding to the burden of her hard work was her constant feeling of needing to prove herself as a good housewife in looking after her husband and her teenage daughter because she felt that she was constantly being judged by her husband's family, who were in the same industry and living close by. Over the previous eight years she had been suffering from panic attacks.

Then four years prior to seeing me she was diagnosed with a myeloproliferative disorder. This is a condition of the bone marrow. She had been fully assessed by a haematologist but refused treatments apart from heparin to thin the blood. She was concerned that the side effects of the treatment would be worse than the condition itself. Also, the proposed treatment would not be curative.

When she first presented, her DASS21 scores were 7–8–13: a moderate level of depression, severe anxiety and severe stress. Because of her busy, hard-working lifestyle, she was not able to attend acupuncture on a weekly basis as I normally recommend but attended for seven sessions over the next 14 weeks.

As you can see from the graph, her scores improved dramatically, all falling to within a normal range in that 14 week period. She attended for a further seven sessions over the next six months and her symptoms of depression, anxiety, and stress all cleared. I followed her up after one year and she assessed her scores as being zero out of 21 in each category. She stated, 'I feel really balanced. I'm allowing life to happen around me and not to me.' This for her was a massive thing because she always felt like it was her job to fix everybody's problems in the house.

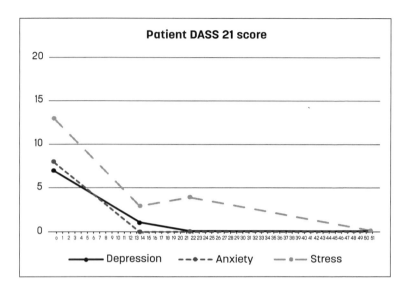

This case illustrates a common phenomenon in depression where there are mixed levels of anxiety and stress together with the depression. It seems that when the depression improves, levels of stress and anxiety also improve dramatically. It also illustrates that Transformational Acupuncture can have a powerful effect, even if it's not given frequently. The case also illustrates that the acupuncture had a beneficial effect on her, despite not having drug therapy or psychological counselling for her depression.

CASE 3:
CHRONIC PAIN FOLLOWING CANCER TREATMENT

An 82-year-old female self-funded retiree

I've been her GP for over 30 years and had always known her to be strong and capable, running her household and finances and always up on current events. She was proud of her independence and saw it as her job to care for her invalid husband and drive him to his appointments.

In 2015, she developed an invasive pharyngeal neoplasm. She had extensive surgery involving the removal of a tonsil, the base of her tongue and the lymph nodes in the right-hand side of her neck. She had follow-up radiotherapy and post-operatively developed a large haematoma in the back of her throat, which required further surgery.

Over the succeeding weeks and months, she had great difficulty swallowing and a constant numbness and burning sensation on the right-hand side of her mouth. Even eight months after surgery she still had chronic pain in the throat with a chronic poor appetite and a chronic dry mouth. The pain was a constant burning sensation. She felt depressed and was frequently waking at night with anxiety attacks.

She was seeing another doctor in the practice who prescribed Panadeine Forte (a paracetamol–codeine combination) and Lyrica (pregabalin) for her neuropathic pain. She was also taking Ativan (lorazepam), an anxiolytic, to help relieve her anxiety attacks, and Endep (amitriptyline), a tricyclic antidepressant. Unfortunately, the medications were not without side effects, causing daytime sleepiness, some dizziness, a slight mental confusion and frequent nausea. She was feeling far from well and looked it. She had a subdued, depressed look on her face. And she was quiet and passive. Normally, she would greet our receptionists in a cheery manner and have a sparkle in her eye. She would usually appear bright and happy, chatting to other patients in the waiting room. Not over the past few months though.

She became totally focused on her symptoms. Her life was falling apart and she felt unable to cope with the smallest problems. Her future looked bleak to her. On many occasions I saw her in the waiting room to see another doctor in the practice and I could see her despair. She kept brushing off my suggestions to try Transformational Acupuncture to alleviate her symptoms as she didn't see it as scientific. After eight months, she gave in and said, 'Okay, I'll try it.' She was at her wits' end. She was having all these medications and getting dizziness, sleepiness and feeling confused and nauseous. She wasn't feeling well at all and she had basically given up any kind of hope. She had no previous history of mental illness apart from rare anxiety attacks.

As she was careful with her money, she agreed to have six treatments over six weeks. As you can see from the DASS score below on the first day, despite all her medications, she was moderately depressed, severely anxious, and moderately stressed. I gave her six sessions of Transformational Acupuncture over six weeks.

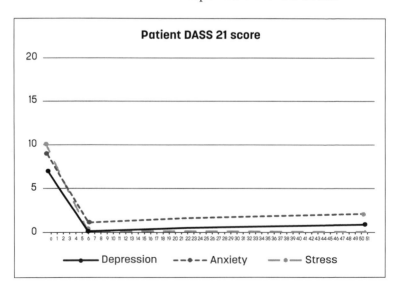

The response was dramatic. She said, 'I'm so much better. I can't believe it myself. My mouth feels better.' She said that there was still a roughness on the right-hand side of her tongue. but it was less sore. As you can see, these results were reflected in the score at week six, which dropped down dramatically to normal levels of depression, anxiety, and stress.

I followed up with her and a year after treatment with acupuncture she is still well, happy, in full control of her life again and caring for her elderly husband. She now only requires a low dose of Lyrica (25mg twice a day compared with 75mg twice a day) to help the abnormal sensation in the mouth, but has not taken any painkillers, antidepressants, or anxiolytics. She hasn't required any acupuncture treatment since.

This case illustrates that a physical illness with potentially life-threatening consequences can certainly affect a person's mind and spirit, as well as their body. The acupuncture helped on all levels. It also demonstrates that the acupuncture worked, despite the patient not having any faith in acupuncture. In fact, she was quite sceptical of it being of any benefit at all. She only submitted to it as she had given up hope that medications were going to help her.

Secondly, this case illustrates that her reactive depression, which was, at 82 years of age, a first episode for her, responded very quickly to acupuncture and the depressed mood has not returned. She continues to be her usual cheerful self with an optimistic outlook on life.

Finally, this case also demonstrates the inadequacies of drug treatment in some instances. The painkillers were not very effective at helping the pain, modestly effective at best. Lyrica did have some benefit in helping dampen the sensations in the mouth but was not without side effects. The dizziness and sleepiness limited the dose she could take. Similarly, she was only taking a low dose of Endep because she couldn't tolerate higher doses of her antidepressant. The anxiolytic relieved the anxiety attacks when they occurred but, of course, did not stop them occurring in the first place. So, the drugs were merely a band-aid treatment rather than a cure. The ongoing symptoms following the surgery and the side effects of the medications were a continual reminder to her that she was not well.

In the real world, drugs often don't seem to work as well as the drug reps and trials would indicate. This raises the issue of the limitations of drug trials and evidence-based medicine in general. When any drug trial is performed, they carefully select who will go into the trial. They don't want any confounding factors. So immediately, elderly people with multiple, complex problems like this patient are excluded.

Incidentally, the young are also excluded from trials. We have generally assumed that antidepressants work as well in adolescents as effectively as adults. Yet the evidence now, some three decades after their introduction into the treatment of depression in adolescents and children, is that antidepressants are no more effective than placebo in treating depression in young people. And more dangerous.

This has been demonstrated in *The Lancet* following a metanalysis of 522 double-blind studies of 21 different antidepressants. Initially, it seemed that fluoxetine was the only antidepressant to be of some benefit in teenagers.[52] A 2019 study funded by the Australian NHMRC concluded that fluoxetine was no more effective than placebo in 15–25 year olds.[53]

Also, drug companies don't want people who are already taking other medications in drug trials. That is understandable as they are trying to standardise the treatment. However, real life is not like that. In the case of this patient, she was elderly and was already taking three other medications before the antidepressant was introduced. Who knows how these drugs would interact with each other – and in an octogenarian? We can't really assume that it will be as safe as giving it to a physically fit and healthy person in their thirties. The evidence is not there.

CASE 4:
A YOUNG WOMAN DEVASTATED BY A DIAGNOSIS OF CANCER

A 37-year-old female cook with two jobs, who at the very young age of 23 developed a malignant melanoma in her arm

The tumour was treated appropriately with a wide excision and then she had a recurrence in the same arm five years later. Again, this was seemingly successfully treated. A year prior to seeing me she felt that she was finally getting her life on track after suffering from several bouts of depression since her teenage years. She had made the decision to separate from her husband, and to quote her, she said, 'I never felt better, happier, or more joyful.'

Unfortunately, this period of happiness was brief. She was devastated six months prior to seeing me to discover that the melanoma had recurred yet again at the age of 36 and metastasised to her axilla. She immediately underwent surgery to remove 17 affected lymph nodes. This was followed up by a course of radiotherapy. She went against medical advice and refused to have chemotherapy as she was concerned about potential side effects.

She said that she had been crying literally daily since the diagnosis of the metastases. She had refused antidepressants offered by her doctor. She had seen a psychologist, but without feeling any benefit. As well as feeling depressed, she also felt chronically tired. She had iron-deficiency anaemia.

As you can see, her DASS scores initially showed severe depression and mild stress without any significant anxiety. A week after her first treatment of Transformational Acupuncture, she said that that was the first week in ages she had gone without crying. She had a total of five sessions over five weeks and stated, 'I feel completely different. My arm feels like a part of my body again.' It was hard for her to describe the feeling, but it was like she had dissociated from her arm. Since the age of 23 she had felt like her arm wasn't a part of her body, but now it did. In fact, she felt so good (as you can see, her scores after five weeks were normal) that she stopped coming for acupuncture.

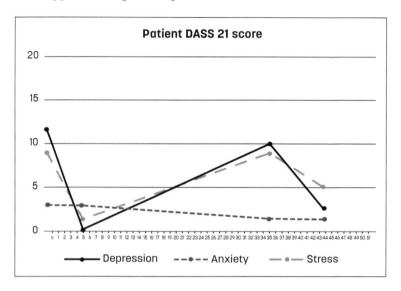

She returned some months later saying, 'I feel almost as bad as before.' The DASS21 score certainly reflects this.

After recommencing Transformational Acupuncture on a fortnightly to three-weekly basis, she said she felt well again. This was reflected in the DASS21 scores coming down to normal. When I followed up with her nearly a year after the initial visit, she said that she felt so well that she had just returned from a six-day 100-kilometre bush walk in Tasmania. And fortunately, she hasn't had any recurrence of her cancer.

This case illustrates that one may present with depression, with or without anxiety. It also illustrates that unless the stressor for the cause of depression is gone, it is important to continue treatment. When a person responds to Transformational Acupuncture, I recommend treatments every three or four weeks as a maintenance for a period of time. Once a person has had regular Transformational Acupuncture, they get a feel for how long the acupuncture effect lasts and can time their visits to suit. If the person can make real changes in their life, they may no longer require acupuncture. I have many patients who come in for a 'top up' on occasions and then go on their way again.

This case also illustrates the connection between mind, body and spirit. From a medical point of view the doctors did their jobs to the best of their ability with surgery and radiotherapy. And this seems to have worked. She has not had a recurrence of her cancer. But it left her feeling damaged. She couldn't describe the sensations, but it felt like her arm didn't belong to her anymore. I do not know if that was due to damage by the radiotherapy to the nerves, or whether it's the psychological issue of feeling like there's a cancerous disease in that arm and her subconscious mind's way of working to try to exclude the cancer was disowning the whole arm. But it's hard to imagine her having real healing unless her arm felt like part of her body again. For this patient Transformational Acupuncture really has been a holistic solution.

CASE 5:
PRESENTED WITH PHYSICAL SYMPTOMS AND
DIDN'T THINK OF HERSELF AS DEPRESSED

A 47-year-old female farmer with a law degree

She presented with an 18-year history of monthly migraine headaches and nausea associated with her periods. Over more recent years she was also suffering from a second kind of headache, cervicogenic headaches – headaches originating from the neck. She found that desk work aggravated her cervicogenic headaches and that painkillers didn't help very much. She was chronically depressed about this.

She had tried various migraine drugs and painkillers, seen a physiotherapist, chiropractor, osteopath, naturopath and a traditional Chinese acupuncturist with no significant or lasting relief.

A couple of years prior to seeing me the patient had also tried Bio-Balance, which is a customised formula of vitamins and minerals based on blood-test results, to improve her mental state. She said it did help to a degree but after a year of taking them daily, she was sick and tired of taking so many tablets and they made her feel nauseous. So, she stopped them about a year prior to seeing me.

She hadn't considered herself depressed, though she described feeling not grounded for four years and described 'inner tension'. She also noted that the headaches seemed worse when her husband was away from home, which with his work was quite frequently. During the few weeks prior to seeing me, she had felt quite stressed about juggling a lot of activities.

The only other significant history was allergic rhinitis, hayfever. She had a dust-mite allergy.

Examination revealed tender, tight neck muscles with some limitation of range of movement, particularly flexion.

Further assessment, using Black Dog Institute's mood assessment program, confirmed that she had non-melancholic depression. Even though this wasn't her presenting problem, it made sense to her that she was feeling depressed. She said she was feeling depressed about getting the headaches, so it became a vicious cycle. That is the depressed mood was causing chronic tension in the head and neck muscles, and the constant pain was making her feel depressed.

As you can see from the graph her initial scores show a moderate level of depression and mild stress.

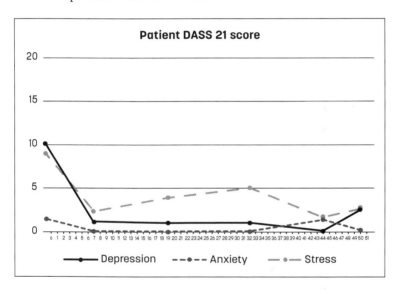

She presented for Transformational Acupuncture on a friend's recommendation. By the end of the first session she said she felt relaxed and that her neck pain had gone. On seeing her a week later, she had remained free of her neck ache and she said she felt a not-unpleasant sensation, 'heavy forehead and eyelids and sinuses, like a releasing sensation'. She also noted 'moments of clarity' that enabled her to make decisions easily.

It was interesting for her to discover during the third session of her Transformational Acupuncture that she became aware of an association between her depressive thoughts and ruminations and the onset of headaches. During the actual session she pulled herself up thinking these depressive thoughts when she could feel the pressure rising in the muscles in her neck and scalp. She immediately let go of those thoughts and the tension eased off straight away.

She completed seven sessions over a period of seven weeks. As you can tell from the seven-week mark on the graph she was no longer feeling depressed or stressed and her levels subsequently remained within the normal range. (The level of stress up to seven is considered normal due to various events happening in people's lives.)

The patient continued coming weekly for a while, until she was free of headaches, and then, as is my usual practice, we stretched the appointments further apart as long as she continued to feel well. The cervicogenic headaches disappeared quickly. The monthly hormonal headaches took a while longer, but they were much less bothersome and didn't require any painkillers.

After a year, she was going for six weeks at a time without any headaches or neck aches and those that she was getting were generally milder and much shorter in duration. Significantly, she could usually identify the trigger on each occasion and take steps to defuse the situation.

The following year this patient consented to be interviewed. These are some excerpts, in which she eloquently describes what her life was like before commencing Transformational Acupuncture and the impact the treatment had on her life:

Dr Alex: What was happening with your daughter and your day-to-day life?

C5:   It got to the point where I was really feeling like I was barely coping. I've got a very supportive husband, but he travels away a lot for work and we live on a farm with our nine-year-old daughter. So, there were times where I was on my own with my daughter and days where I probably had to get her to make her own lunch. And then I'd get out of bed and take her to school, come back home and go to bed. And then wake up, pick her up from school. And make sure her needs were met, and the animals, and things like that, but then was heading back to bed again. So, there were days like that that were really, really difficult. And they were happening quite a lot.

I had to really get back to basics and just do the bare minimum. I had to cut back on my engagement with the school and how much I could do on the farm. I started to really feel like my mental state, my mood, was really suffering because of the painful headaches and because of my inability to be involved and do all this stuff that I was used to doing.

Dr Alex: Can you tell us a little bit about your first treatment?

C5: Yes, so I had been in more pain at that time, a lot of chronic headaches, four or five days a week. And I just remember that first treatment felt like a bit of a circuit-breaker actually. It was instantaneous; it was very relaxing. I felt a really strong release of tension in my head, and in my neck. That lasted probably for a good couple of days afterwards. So, I did feel a strong effect after that first treatment, definitely.

Dr Alex: Oh, excellent. Can you tell us some of the changes that you've experienced as a result of coming for acupuncture of the past twelve months?

C5: Of course. The following acupuncture treatments were very relaxing. I found an improvement in my headaches, definitely, quite quickly. Sometimes I did feel like it was two steps forward, one step back, in that I was still getting headaches, but generally, I was doing much better. I came to realise, I guess after a number of months, that there was this really powerfully cumulative effect in these treatments that was building over time. So, I got some great results early on. But I was really starting to notice this really longer-lasting cumulative effect of the ongoing treatments.

Dr Alex: That's great. Patients often comment on that cumulative effect over time. Can you tell us about some of the changes that you've made in your life?

C5: I'm generally much more positive about life. I feel like I've got more in my tank, so to speak. I'm not in that chronic-headache place anymore, which is fantastic. I still get some headaches, but they're much shorter in duration and much milder. So that's given me a lot of space in my life to kind of think of other things. I have periods where I feel much better. I feel much lighter and have more clarity around my thinking. I'm generally more hopeful about life, and more engaged with my community and my daughter's school. I feel much more excited about getting back into that kind of thing, which is really good.

Dr Alex: And you started a new project. What's that?

C5: It came as a really big surprise, to me even. But late last year, I started writing a blog, which is something I never thought I would ever do. But I have to say it's been fantastic and I doubt whether I would have even realised that it was something that I wanted to do, let alone have had the courage to do it, if I hadn't gone through this process of treatment. So, Transformational Acupuncture did more than relieve pain, it gave me this, I guess, space in my own mind to explore a whole lot of other things, which is terrific.

Dr Alex: Yes! And you've come to some insights around your condition and health and things. Can you share some of those?

C5: I have. Sure. On reflection, I realised that I guess I was thinking a lot about my condition purely as a physical condition. I guess the biggest realisation I've had is that my condition is as much about my mental health, as it is my physical health. I've realised that these acupuncture treatments have probably been dealing with both of those elements, which the other treatments weren't dealing with as much. So, I feel like the acupuncture has really kind of settled my nervous system down, and it's had a really fantastic effect on what's going on in my body, but it's really helped me with a whole lot of underlying issues. I've realised I've had some anxieties, stress and overthinking. Transformational Acupuncture has had a really profound effect on my emotional and mental state. And I think that has been the big thing for me actually. It's made the big difference in this treatment, as it's very holistic.

Dr Alex: Thank you for sharing. Is there anything else you would like to mention?

C5: Yes, just reflecting on these realisations. You see I've had acupuncture before, the traditional Chinese medicine-type acupuncture. It was very helpful in relieving the headaches, but short-term only. The difference with the Transformational Acupuncture for me is this cumulative effect that it's had and the effect on my general overall mental wellbeing. I think it's a really wonderful holistic type of acupuncture. I think it's quite different to any other acupuncture I've had before.

Over a period of a few months, her attitude to life changed completely. Her blogging was very successful. She followed this up by attending a creative writing workshop in the United States.

After discussions with her husband, she realised that she wasn't so attached to her farm or the rural town where she lived. Ultimately, she, her husband and daughter moved to Europe. She now has a very creative job as a project manager for a large, international non-profit organisation. She also has a very active social life with her husband, attending concerts and sight-seeing.

The contrast with isolated living on a farm and barely surviving the day, with a frequently absent husband, couldn't be greater.

This case illustrates that often patients don't present with mental-health problems. Instead they are often focused on their physical symptoms. In this case, headaches. That was the issue that drove her to seek help. It was her body's way of indicating to her that there was a problem.

Secondly, it also illustrates that there is a concomitant improvement in symptoms of physical problems as well as mental problems with Transformational Acupuncture. Despite modern medicine's efforts toward ever more specialist treatment, it is impossible to separate mind, body and spirit. In this case, her lack of fulfillment and general dissatisfaction with her life and her feeling of impotence in not being able do anything about it led to a feeling of being down and ruminating on what to do. This in turn manifested in continual muscle tension and hormonal imbalance, resulting in her headaches.

Thirdly, it illustrates that often people who are depressed feel stuck. They don't see any solutions or see the bigger picture. So, they are unable to come up with solutions to change the circumstances in their life. I believe Transformational Acupuncture was instrumental in giving her clarity of mind to have these realisations, make decisions and take action to turn her dreams into reality. Her life has been completely transformed. The headaches and depressed feelings are a thing of the past.

9

CHANGING THE PSYCHOLOGY OF DEPRESSION – WHAT CAN I DO TO HELP MYSELF

'What can I do to help myself?' I hear you ask. That is a great question, for a start. It is a great question because it gets you in the frame of mind for seeking answers. I think it is the first step on the road to recovery. It is a much more positive question than, 'Why does this always happen to me?' or 'Why doesn't anyone like me?' To answer the question of what you can do to help yourself it helps to use the Cognitive Behaviour Therapy (CBT) model of change.

THE INTERPLAY BETWEEN THOUGHTS, FEELINGS, BEHAVIOUR AND THE PHYSICAL BODY

THE CBT MODEL

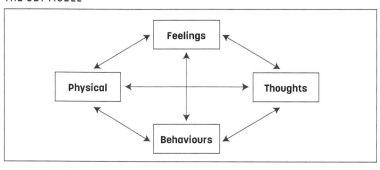

Source: RACGP gplearning

The CBT model sees an interplay between your thoughts, feelings and behaviour and connects these with the physical aspect of your being. In depression, people can become stuck in a negative feedback where their thoughts, feelings, behaviour and physiological state conspire to keep you stuck in a black hole.

THE CBT MODEL IN ACTION

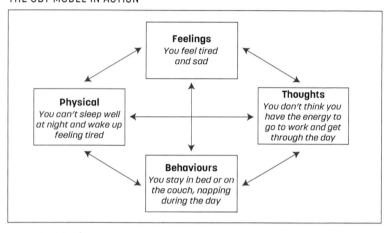

Source: RACGP gplearning

For example, in this model we see the individual is *feeling* tired and sad. This impacts the person's *behaviour* by staying in bed or lying on the couch and falling asleep in front of the PlayStation. They have the *thought* that they don't have the energy to go to work or even get through the day. They don't even want to leave the house. In a *physical* sense, they decondition, don't sleep well at night and wake up feeling tired. These all feed back into each other. The person feels stuck and helpless, a victim of their circumstances.

Exercise and diet

Change any one of these, and it will have an influence on the other aspects. For example, set an alarm, get out of bed, and put on jogging gear left out the night before and go for a walk. Of course, doing this once won't have a lasting effect. But doing it day after day will. It will become a new behaviour, a habit. It will start changing you physically, losing weight and strengthening muscles. You'll start to feel energised and, dare I say it, happier. Couple this with focussing your mind on things that you can be grateful for in your life, and day by day you will change your life. This sounds simplistic. But it can work.

I had a patient who did this, without any prompting from me. Her sister challenged her to run with her later in the year at Sydney's annual City2Surf 14km fun run. Despite a lifetime of inactivity, she started with setting a target of walking 10,000 steps each morning; then made progress with a couch-to-10k phone app. In the process she ended up losing 30kg and became much fitter. It made her think twice about eating comfort foods. It completely changed her mindset, her view of herself and her understanding of what was possible. Needless to say, she no longer feels depressed and like a helpless victim of her circumstances. Her outlook on life has completely changed. Now she and her sister regularly run in marathons.

Another approach could be to focus on changing your diet. What you put in your mouth can influence your mood. Reducing processed foods, especially "junk food" and having more fresh fruit and vegetables, fish and whole grains has been demonstrated in an Australian study to improve the symptoms of major depressive disorder.[54] In another Australian study, depression scores improved into the normal range in just *three weeks* on such a diet.[55] It is thought that improving the diet has an anti-inflammatory effect on the brain, as well as the rest of the body. Or rather, that eating a diet full of junk food is pro-inflammatory. It literally irritates the brain.

Gratitude and meditation

Of course, these are just two ways of making a change. Adjusting your exercise routine and diet results in physical changes that impact your physiological state, but you can also initiate change by changing your thoughts. As I mentioned in the earlier example, you can start just by thinking about things you can be grateful for. This is focussing on some of the positive things in your life and the world around you rather than what you see as being wrong with your life or the world. Try this in combination with exercise, such as going for a walk; however, if you find this difficult you could also try journaling. This can be as simple as writing down something positive that happened in your day. Day by day this simple list will grow. At times when you are down and life seems bleak, you can review your list and realise that your life isn't a total disaster, that positive things do happen. By regularly being grateful for the small things in life, I think you can develop an attitude of gratitude.

Another way of changing your thoughts is to spend time each day meditating. This basically involves quietening the body, quietening the mind and just observing what is going on inside you. There are many free guided meditations available online or on smartphone apps that can get you started. This practice can also be combined with yoga, which has the added benefit of bringing mind and body together as it works on changing your physiological state.

Another approach to making change is by keeping a track of your feelings and trying to observe common situations that regularly trigger certain emotions. This is best done with a mood tracking app, of which there are numerous available for your smartphone.

Counselling
Making changes in all these aspects of thoughts, feelings, behaviours and physiology can have a huge impact on improving your mental health, but it is easy to feel overwhelmed and scattered trying to make too many changes at once. My suggestion is to start with the method that sounds most attractive to you, whether it is going for a walk each morning, or sitting meditating or changing your diet.

And that brings us to the heart of the problem of depression. When you are in a state of depression it is hard enough to get through the day, let alone commit to all of these activities which take conscious effort and focus, each and every day. A counsellor can be invaluable to help keep you on track and focussed on your goals, as well as help you sort out your feelings and thoughts. This could be a trained psychologist or a trusted friend or buddy.

All this said, sometimes we need immediate support. If you or someone you know are in crisis, call 000 or one of the following Australian helplines for help:

>   Lifeline Australia – 13 11 14
>   Suicide Call Back Service – 1300 659 467

For those not in immediate crisis or danger, a wealth of resources and fact sheets – including self-assessments for depression, anxiety and bipolar disorder – are available from the Black Dog Institute: www.blackdoginstitute.org.au.

Beyond Blue also provides a range of useful resources, helpfully categorised by age, gender, and ethnicity: www.beyondblue.org.au.

Medication

Antidepressants may very well be necessary. I am not against anti-depressants, just the indiscriminate use of antidepressants. I think antidepressants help depression primarily by affecting feelings. They dampen down feelings of sadness, despair and hopelessness. But, unfortunately, I think they blunt feelings of joy and happiness as well. For the severely depressed, this may be necessary, but this limits the benefits for the mildly depressed. Medication may influence the physiology in making a person feel calmer and less tense, but this usually accompanied by lethargy and tiredness. Also, the drugs won't directly change thoughts or behaviours. So alone, antidepressant drugs aren't the total answer.

Acupuncture

This is where I feel acupuncture has a huge role to play. I think it works on all levels of changing the physiology, the feelings, the thoughts and ultimately the behaviour. Apart from taking medication, all the other methods I've discussed require conscious effort on the part of the patient. Acupuncture does not – apart from turning up for the weekly session. I saw this clearly with Chewie, the patient I mentioned in the preface. I was shocked when I first saw him for acupuncture. I had known him as a gregarious, life-of-the-party family man. The day he was brought in by his wife for his first treatment, he looked dull and lifeless. There was no spark or twinkle in his eyes. He spoke in monosyllables. It was all he could do to turn up each week, but he seemed to come to life after about the third or fourth session. By the eighth session, he seemed back to his usual self and was able to speak eloquently about how he got into such a depressed state and what the journey had been like for him.

I think acupuncture affects the physiology by switching off the sympathetic nervous system. Often depressed people are in a hypervigilant state. They are constantly anxious and stressed. Patients typically comment that they feel calmer and more relaxed, even by the end of the first treatment.

Acupuncture seems to directly affect a patient's thoughts. Brooke, a 39-year-old mother and wife, has been attending on a monthly basis for a long period of time for post-traumatic stress disorder following sexual abuse as a child. Together with psychological counselling, acupuncture helped her go through with taking the matter to the police, deal with the ensuing court case in which the perpetrator was sentenced to several years' jail and cope with the fallout from those who felt she was to blame for destroying their family. She stated that she keeps coming back for acupuncture because, 'I always get good advice'. She didn't mean me; she meant the thoughts that came to mind!

Acupuncture decreases the chatter of the monkey mind and allows deep and meaningful thoughts to come to the fore. It would normally take months of practising daily meditation for this to happen. One 43-year-old lady with a moderate level of chronic depression commented at the end of her very first acupuncture session, 'I was surprised. All these positive thoughts came through.' Another patient, Jill, commented after the third session, 'Funny, but I've noticed all that internal dialogue quieten right down.' Bill said, 'It was strange. I know I was awake, but I wasn't thinking of anything.' I think these are examples of mindfulness, and they develop spontaneously during the acupuncture session.

I caution that not all patients are suitable to undergo this kind of acupuncture. It requires courage sometimes to process these thoughts. One patient, Ellen, during her third treatment had a sudden emotional release of tears. She stopped coming for acupuncture after that. Many years later told me that she had stopped coming because 'I was on the verge of remembering something I didn't want to remember'.

Patients often tell me emotions are released during the acupuncture, or in the few days after a session. It usually results from suppressed emotions: for example, grief associated with unresolved mourning, and buried anger and frustration may be expressed. This can be shocking for the patient as well as for the person on the receiving end. The patient always feels better after. I think patients handle this better when forewarned. If meltdowns are going to happen, it is usually early in the course of treatments and typically only happens once.

In summary, I think patients with enquiring minds and insight do much better with acupuncture (and counselling) than someone who just wants the bad feelings to go away.

10

ACUPUNCTURE FAQS

Patients and doctors alike often ask me a wide variety of questions about acupuncture, and these are some of the most common ones. Especially if you have never had acupuncture before, it is worth reading these FAQs. Some people who try acupuncture for the first time are quite shocked at the effect that it can have on them. It isn't always pleasant and relaxing, though it usually is. If you know what to expect it will help you to 'go with the flow' of the changes that the treatment has on you, and I think that this knowledge will help expedite the change.

GENERAL INFORMATION

Q: How does acupuncture work?
A: That's a good question. It's not totally known how acupuncture works. But what we do know is, you put a needle in and it creates a sensation; it's stimulating the nerve endings under the skin and in the muscles, which give the sensation of what's called proprioception, the awareness of position and movement of the body. If you close your eyes, you know where your hands and feet are without having to look, and that's because you've got this sense

in the body that knows where all your parts are. So, it seems to be stimulating those nerves particularly. In the spinal cord, where there are synapses, or nerves, joined from one to the next, and the signals are long, acupuncture seems to block C fibres particularly. C fibres are fibres that carry pain signals, so acupuncture alters the perception of pain, and dulls it. And after several treatments it can actually switch off the pain signals.

Secondly, acupuncture has been shown to affect the levels of various neurotransmitters, or chemical messengers in the synapses or connections, between nerve cells in the brain and spinal cord as well as the peripheral nerves. Acupuncture seems to *enhance* the activity of:

- endogenous opioid peptides (morphine-like)
- serotonin (the happy chemical)
- dopamine (involved in addictive behaviour, and lacking in Parkinson's disease)
- acetylcholine (especially found in the parasympathetic nervous system, which calms and nurtures the body)
- gamma-aminobutyric acid (GABA, the body's natural Valium)
- glycine (affects mood, cognition, memory, learning, appetite and sleep)
- taurine (anti-anxiety, antidepressant effects)

It also seems to *attenuate* the activity of:

- norepinephrine (noradrenaline, puts the brain in a state of heightened arousal)
- glutamate (an excitatory neurotransmitter)
- aspartate (another excitatory neurotransmitter).[56]

Thirdly, various acupuncture points can stimulate the release of various hormones from the endocrine glands and various chemicals from the exocrine glands.

Acupuncture has been demonstrated to affect the blood levels in humans of the following hormones:

- oestradiol (E2),
- follicular stimulating hormone (FSH)
- luteinising hormone (LH)
- progesterone
- prolactin
- gonadotrophin releasing hormone (GnRH)
- human chorionic gonadotrophin (hCG)
- oxytocin
- cortisol.[57] [58]

In rat experiments, acupuncture has been demonstrated to affect the hypothalamus–pituitary–adrenal axis, the hypothalamus–pituitary–thyroid axis and the hypothalamus–pituitary–gonadal axis.[59]

The autonomic nervous system controls all the endocrine glands, which are the glands that release hormones into the bloodstream. Acupuncture works directly through the peripheral nervous system to feedback to the brain to alter brain function. For example, Dr Im Quah-Smith, of Sydney, Australia, performed a study where she needled a point near the knee that has been known in Chinese medicine for a couple of thousand years to affect liver function. Dr Quah-Smith was able to demonstrate that when she needled that particular point, a certain area in the brain lit up on an MRI scan, and simultaneously resulted in increased blood flow to the liver.

Given that there are 361 standard acupuncture points affecting various organ functions in various ways, I think it's incredibly complex and exciting to discover how these things work.

Q: Isn't acupuncture just an elaborate placebo?

A: Acupuncturists are doing acupuncture because they get results. I don't think that it is credible to believe that acupuncturists are charlatans and quacks. I know I wouldn't be performing acupuncture if I didn't believe it was working. And I'm sure my patients wouldn't be paying good money if they didn't believe it was working either.

Q: How many treatments does it take before I see an improvement in my mental health?

A: Acupuncture patients generally fall into three groups. The first group is the majority of patients, probably around 60–70 per cent. They report improvement in symptoms within three or four treatments. The benefits usually last a day or two, then the symptoms return to the level they had before the acupuncture. Sometimes the improvement lasts only a few hours. But even so, if it only lasts a few hours after the first treatment this is a good sign. I find that the benefits last longer and longer with subsequent treatments, until the relief of symptoms last until the next visit. I then stretch out the appointments from weekly to fortnightly, fortnightly to every third week, and so on.

Some patients respond to the acupuncture dramatically on the first time. Recently, I had a 67-year-old male patient, Tony, diagnosed with benign paroxysmal positional vertigo. He had the vertigo daily for over three months. No treatment from the ear, nose and throat surgeon or GP helped. A week after that first treatment he happily reported that the symptoms disappeared with the first session of acupuncture. I have given him two further weekly treatments. He is still asymptomatic, and very happy.

Another patient 64-year-old female, Danielle, who unfortunately has rectal cancer which has metastasised to her liver and lungs. She came to me because she developed a peripheral neuropathy as a side effect of the chemotherapy. She had the symptoms continuously for seven months. She described her feet as feeling icy and having twitching toes. Her ankles felt puffy. She had milder symptoms in her hands. By the time I inserted the fifth acupuncture needle in her during the first treatment she reported that the twitching feeling had stopped, after experiencing it constantly for many months! By the end of the treatment her feet felt less icy, and her hands felt normal. Most of the benefit lasted until I saw her for her second treatment a week later. As a doctor I feel very heartened and encouraged by these stories, because as you know patients generally don't do well with medical treatment for these conditions. These patients don't have to suffer these symptoms. I always encourage patients to try acupuncture because you never know how much they may benefit, and the risk is minimal.

I have found that patients can sometimes be enthusiastic at first about acupuncture, but after a few treatments state that the acupuncture isn't helping. I have found that usually within three or four treatments I get a feel for how the patient is going with acupuncture. Quite often it is obvious to me as well as the patient themselves whether or not they are responding well to treatment.

If they show no change after some 6–8 weekly sessions, then I advise them to try something else for their problem. I don't string the patient along and I don't think other acupuncturists would either. When the patient continually reports no change in symptoms, they are considered non-responders to acupuncture. This probably accounts for 20 per cent of those trying acupuncture.

There is a smaller subsection, who seem like non-responders, and only start noticing an improvement in symptoms after more than three or four sessions. Generally, I will give patients the benefit of the doubt for eight sessions over eight weeks. For example, Monica, a 54-year-old female, presented to me with severe depression. Her DASS score was 14–10–16, very high, despite being on Lexapro (escitalopram), an antidepressant, 20mg 1½ daily; Zyprexa (olanzapine), an antipsychotic given to sedate;

and Xanax (alprazolam), an anxiolytic, 1mg in the morning and
½ at midday. She had very blunted affect, in that she showed little
emotion. She came weekly. Each time she reported that she was
'still anxious' and 'no change' in her symptoms, that the acupuncture did 'nothing really'. She said this for seven treatments, then
was admitted by her psychiatrist to the psychiatric unit for seven
weeks. During this time, her medication was changed to Efexor
(venlafaxine), an antidepressant, 337.5mg in the morning; Lyrica
(pregabalin), an anticonvulsant that decreases chronic pain,
125mg twice a day; and Rivotril (clonazepam), an anxiolytic,
0.5mg in the morning. When I saw her after being discharged
her DASS score was still a disappointing 12–12–15. She still
had a blunt affect. Her voice was a monotone and her face was
expressionless. She was still a woman of few words and was still
complaining of anxiety. I recommended weekly acupuncture, but
she continually said that she felt 'nothing really'. When I came into
remove the acupuncture needles at the end of the seventh session
of the second round of treatments, you could have knocked me
down with a feather. I went into the room and she was laughing
and smiling. The next time I saw her she reported that she was
'not too bad'. The time after, she said, 'I'm feeling quite good.' At
the end of the tenth session, she said, 'I'm happy as Larry!' And
she looked it.

Interestingly, a group of patients, probably around 10 per
cent, will find that the acupuncture stirs up the symptoms, for
a few days. I don't tell these patients acupuncture isn't working
but encourage them to return for further treatment. These are
definitely worth pursuing, as it means the acupuncture is working.
I just space the treatments further apart. After the initial flare up
of symptoms, if one waits long enough there is a period when
the symptoms settle to a point below what they had before the
treatment. In these cases, I will modify what acupuncture points I
am using and treat them once every three weeks instead. Over time

these patients usually do well. I have often noticed this situation in patients with chronic fatigue syndrome or fibromyalgia associated with their depression. They can feel wiped out for a few days after acupuncture. I have learned to do gentle treatments at first and wait longer between treatments.

Q: Why is it so difficult to prove that acupuncture works?

A: As you may appreciate, the hard evidence is difficult to come by. There are a number of reasons for this. Not the least is that lack of resources to study acupuncture. Drug companies can afford to run multimillion-dollar trials. Patenting a successful drug will give the company exclusive rights to worldwide sales for the next dozen or so years. This amounts to billions of dollars. This is not possible with acupuncture. There is no pot of gold at the end of an acupuncture trial, so there is no large corporate backing. It is not easy to perform acupuncture trials in the large numbers and the length of time needed to demonstrate a clear effect with limited resources.

A second important reason is the difficulty blinding the patient and the acupuncturist. It is difficult to fool a patient as to whether they are having a needle stuck in them or not. And how can an acupuncturist be blinded to whether they are performing acupuncture or not? By contrast, it is a fairly simple matter to compare a drug with a placebo tablet.

Thirdly, most of the acupuncture trials are performed in China, backed by a government that does have the resources to sponsor acupuncture trials. Criticism from the West surrounds the lack of a placebo arm in these trials. The Chinese have a different mindset. For them it is unethical to give a treatment that they think won't work, a placebo. Outcomes from these trials are automatically dismissed by the West, and these medical authorities conclude that there is no evidence acupuncture works.

Q: Is there evidence that acupuncture works?

A: In the past handful of years, good quality trials have been published to demonstrate its effectiveness. Go to The Acupuncture Evidence Project web page for a summary of evidence for its effectiveness in a number of medical conditions: www.acupuncture. org.au/resources/publications/the-acupuncture-evidence-project

There is a plain-English summary of medical conditions that may be helped by acupuncture. This was published in February 2017.

Q: Is all acupuncture the same, or are there different types?

A: There are many schools of thought, methods and techniques of acupuncture that have been developed over the centuries. The most widespread and original is the acupuncture that came out of China based on the past couple of millennia of traditional Chinese medicine. Japanese acupuncture and Korean acupuncture also have a lengthy history. There are various other recent systems like auriculotherapy, ear acupuncture, from France. Even within traditional Chinese acupuncture there are various schools based on the teachings of various masters. All these systems seem to have their strengths and weaknesses.

Q: What is the difference between Transformational Acupuncture and other forms of acupuncture?

A: I recently developed Transformational Acupuncture, based on the works of Dr Mikio Sankey, established in 1997, which in turn is based on traditional Chinese acupuncture together with the Indian Ayurvedic understanding of the body. The technique involved is similar to Japanese acupuncture in that the gentle Japanese-type needles are used, and the insertion is fairly shallow. Most Australians find this kind of acupuncture more acceptable than Chinese acupuncture, which uses thicker, rougher needles, which are inserted deeper, and are often stimulated – that is, the acupuncturist twirls or lifts and thrusts the needle to create a stronger sensation. Some people enjoy that effect and feel it is giving them a good, strong treatment. However, most patients I have much prefer the gentler technique! Transformational Acupuncture is very gentle. Often people don't even notice or feel the needle insertion, and yet it can have a deep, profound effect on the psyche as well as the body.

Q: Is Transformational Acupuncture recognised by the medical profession?
A: Acupuncture is recognised by the medical community as safe and effective. I think most of the medical profession would be unaware of the various types of acupuncture systems that are available, however. I have branded the Transformational Acupuncture System because it is a specific system with defined protocols that has a demonstrated effect in a randomised, controlled setting.

THE PROCEDURE

Q: Are there any side effects with acupuncture?
A: Generally, acupuncture is amazingly side-effect free. Bruising can occur sometimes. Potentially acupuncture could have significant side effects, like puncturing a lung or so forth, but that is incredibly rare. Only ninety deaths have been noted in modern times, despite millions upon millions of acupuncture treatments.

In Transformational Acupuncture, the needling is superficial, which should make the risk of this unlikely side effect non-existent. Compare this with Dr Peter Gøtzsche's claims that psychiatric drugs are responsible for more than half a million deaths in over-65 year olds each and every year.[60]

Q: Will acupuncture hurt?
A: Generally, there's much less discomfort or pain involved than most people think. After their first treatment, most people who

haven't had acupuncture before say, 'Oh, is that all there is to it? It doesn't hurt like I was expecting.' But, on the other hand, sometimes some patients can feel quite strong sensations on some points. The more out of balance the energy is at a point, the more you will feel it. It's the muscles with the knots that feel painful and uncomfortable when being massaged. And yet, at the same time, you don't want the massage therapist to stop because that feels good. I think it is something similar with acupuncture. In the Transformational Acupuncture System, Japanese-style needles are used. These are finer and smoother than traditional Chinese needles, and thus cause less sensation when inserted.

Also, the insertion is relatively superficial, which again means less sensation. Further, once inserted the needles are left alone. There is no twirling and rotating, and there is no lifting and thrusting. So again, there is less sensation than Chinese techniques.

Q: Will I be sore after acupuncture?

A: Generally, no. Most people will feel more energised and more alert after a treatment. Often, pain conditions can feel a lot less painful immediately after the treatment has finished.

Sometimes, however, acupuncture can 'stir things up' and give a general feeling of achiness, which can come on a few hours after the treatment, but usually resolves within 24–48 hours. I think this is like the effect of a deep-tissue massage, which can leave you feeling a bit fluey or unwell for a few hours to a day or two after treatment as it's shifting things. This might happen once or twice during a course of treatments if there is a big shift of energy. The person usually feels much better after that.

NEEDLES

Q: What if I have a needle phobia?

A: Well, if a person has a needle phobia I start off very gently and very slowly. I use needles that I would use on children to produce minimal sensation. Often, I'll say, 'Just let me put the first needle in and see how you feel.' And once people have the needle they say, 'Oh, that's okay.' I ask them, 'Did you feel that?' And they usually say, 'No, not really.' And then I'll encourage them with the second needle.

With children, I often will start by using laser acupuncture. That produces a beam of laser light so there is absolutely no sensation involved, let alone pain or discomfort. And once I gain their trust and they feel confident that the laser works, I'll ask them if I can try just one needle and laser the rest of the points.

After a few sessions, most children over the age of seven will be quite happy with needle acupuncture as they know they will feel very good in a short while. In fact, most children will leave the clinic with a smile on their face.

Q: Do the same needles get reused?

A: No, in Australia acupuncture needles are sterile, are single-use only and are disposed of in the appropriate manner in sharps containers. So, there is no chance of transmitting infections from one person to another.

Q: Are there any chemicals in acupuncture needles?

A: No. The needles are solid stainless steel. It is possible to have silver or gold needles, but for obvious reasons these are rarely used!

Q: Are the needles inserted in the same place each time?

A: The treatments are personalised in that where the needles are placed depends on the energy blocks. Some people will need the same treatment repeated a few times to shift a certain blockage. Quite often the needles are placed in a different place every time as the condition shifts and improves.

Q: If I have an injury, will the needles be placed in the injury site?
A: Generally, no. Acupuncture works through stimulating the nervous system. Given that acupuncture works based on the channels or meridians in the body, one can influence an injured area while placing the needle some distance away from that area.

Also, it is not recommended to insert a needle into diseased or broken skin, or close to a fracture, because of the concern of introducing infection into the body.

Q: Why do I feel a strange sensation in a different place to the acupuncture site?
A: That's another good question. Often people will say, 'Oh, did you put a needle in my …' and name a part of their body away from the acupuncture site. And I'll say, 'No, there's no needles anywhere near it.' Yet to them it felt like there was a needle there. I think this is because the area they may have felt some sensation was where the energy was getting blocked and the acupuncture was trying to shift the blockage in that channel.

Often people will report various strange sensations. It can make one limb feel larger than the other one. It can make it feel like the head is on back to front. It can give people a sensation of gentle rocking and floating on water. Sometimes it gives a feeling of being incredibly heavy, yet at other times it gives a feeling of being light and floating, often in the same person and often even in the same acupuncture session. People sometimes swear the door has moved to the other side of the room from where they came in. I think this is because the acupuncture is influencing the nerves for proprioception. Proprioception is our ability to know our body's position in space.

I think it's marvellous how acupuncture stimulates the nervous system in ways that we haven't even probably thought about.

Q: Will acupuncture make me bleed?

A: Generally, no. Acupuncture needles are very fine, around twice the diameter of a human hair and have a blunt, rounded end rather than a sharp point. As the needle is being inserted, the blunt end tends to push blood vessels to one side or the other rather than cutting them like a needle used for collecting blood or doing pathology tests which will have a sharp, bevelled edge. This means that there is no bleeding when an acupuncture needle is withdrawn.

However, if the area is congested there will often be a drop of blood and there may be a small bruise, but usually not anything more than that. Even for people on blood-thinning drugs, it still doesn't seem to make them bleed or bruise any more than normal. If they are on warfarin and their INR (a measure of how thick the blood is) is greater than 2.5, that could possibly result in more significant bruising. But in my experience, I haven't really found this to be a problem.

ACUPUNCTURE AND MEDICAL CONDITIONS

Q: What conditions can be helped by acupuncture?

A: Acupuncture can be used to help a huge variety of conditions. Firstly, it is important to realise that it won't make any medical problem worse. Furthermore, there are no adverse effects from using it as an adjunct to modern medical drug treatments or surgical procedures. I've used it for a wide variety of medical problems.

Other than mental-health problems, which have been detailed in this book, I have used it for acute pain conditions, such as injuries, as well as for chronic pain conditions, such as chronic back pain, arthritis pain, period pain, migraine headaches and tension headaches. In most cases pain is eased or relieved.

However, use of opioid painkillers such as oxycodone (OxyContin) and anxiolytic benzodiazepines such as diazepam (Valium) tend to weaken the effect of acupuncture. Patience is required when patients are taking these sorts of drugs in high doses. Generally, acupuncture will help them, but will take longer to work. I have used acupuncture to help when there are autonomic nervous system dysfunctions – that is, where there is an imbalance between the sympathetic and parasympathetic nervous systems, such as asthma, heart palpitations, irritable bowel syndrome, indigestion of various kinds, and so forth. For a more complete list see: www.acupuncture.org.au/resources/publications/the-acupuncture-evidence-project

Q: Does acupuncture help with the side effects of chemotherapy?
A: Please note that I would never claim acupuncture is an alternative treatment to Western medicine with cancer, but it is a useful adjunct. It generally helps the nausea, listlessness and weakness that people often have when they are receiving chemotherapy. This makes the chemotherapy better tolerated. Our local oncologist is happy enough for me to perform acupuncture on cancer patients as it does not interfere with any of the chemotherapy drugs, unlike herbs of Chinese or Western varieties and megadoses of vitamins.

Q: Can I have acupuncture while pregnant?
A: Depending on the pregnancy-related symptoms one is treating, yes. There are some points in Chinese medicine that should not be used during pregnancy, but acupuncture can work very well with symptoms of morning sickness, low-back pain, pelvic pain and other problems of pregnancy.

Q: Will acupuncture help balance my hormones?

A: I think acupuncture has an enormous effect on hormone levels. The whole of Chinese philosophy is based on yin–yang and the idea of finding balance. This is a model of homeostasis that is comparable, I think, to the sympathetic and parasympathetic nervous system, which innervates all the organs in the body, including the endocrine organs that produce hormones.

Q: If someone is already taking antidepressants, is having acupuncture at the same time possible?

A: Absolutely. Acupuncture doesn't interfere with antidepressants and vice versa. In fact, if anything, there's a synergistic effect. That is, they help one another. Particularly SSRIs. One of the effects of antidepressants is thought to be that they prevent the re-uptake of serotonin (a neurotransmitter) at the synapse (or nerve junction). Antidepressants haven't been demonstrated to increase overall levels of serotonin. Whereas, studies have shown that acupuncture actually increases the production of serotonin. For example, a 2015 clinical study demonstrated that serum levels of 5 hydroxytryptamine (5-HT), also known as serotonin rose, after treatment with acupuncture for depression. At the same time levels of interleukin-6 (IL-6), a marker for inflammation, actually decreased.[61]

It seems logical to me that if acupuncture is increasing the production of serotonin, it's actually going to make the anti-depressants more effective at utilising serotonin.

Q: Can acupuncture be used instead of medication for depression?

A: During our acupuncture trial for depression we found that a number of patients have been able to reduce or get off anti-depressants. My first case where a patient was able to cease antidepressants was back in 2013. I saw a lady who had been on antidepressants for 16 years, and I was treating her for her osteo-arthritis. Over the space of a couple of months, she was able to get off the antidepressants because she felt so well, calm and relaxed because of the acupuncture. She has not needed to resort to any antidepressants, or painkillers for that matter, since then.

However, I caution against patients taking matters into their own hands and stopping their medication. A lot of antidepressants must be weaned. One can't suddenly stop them because of the side effects of withdrawal, so-called discontinuation syndrome. The patient must be monitored by their medical practitioner. So, any reduction or stopping of antidepressant medication should only be done under medical advice. And it's possible to do this by monitoring with DASS scores and similar scales of measuring mental health or mental stress.

It's interesting that I've always had a passion, I guess, for de-prescribing. De-prescribing is a new buzzword in the medical world and refers to withdrawing people from medications, particularly the elderly in nursing homes. It is not uncommon for patients to be on 20+ different medications, each taken several times a day. Who would know the potential interactions between all those drugs, whether all those drugs are necessary? So, there is a process now of reviewing medication and gradually withdrawing all the unnecessary ones to simplify treatment. Even as a hospital intern forty years ago, I always took delight in being able to stop patient's medications in hospital. (I'm sure some of my colleagues at the time thought it was perverse delight!) It was the process of seeing people recover and getting better to the point where they didn't need the medications anymore. I felt that I was helping them on the road to full independence again.

Maybe part of why I find acupuncture such a thrilling method to use is because it can help people to de-prescribe. It is safe and effective, and people are quite frequently able to be withdrawn from various medications including antidepressants, anxiolytics, sleeping tablets and painkillers, which are a huge burden on society, besides the obvious economic burden.

Q: Can it help chronic pain?

A: Unlike painkillers, acupuncture is not actually masking the pain. I think it switches off the pain process, the signals going from the body up to the brain. As it is switching off pain centres in the brain, this makes it very useful for neuropathic pain. This is the kind of pain that occurs for months after an attack of shingles and also in trigeminal neuralgia. These types of painful conditions can be difficult to treat medically and the drugs used can have significant side effects, so I get a great sense of satisfaction helping people with these debilitating conditions.

THE EFFECTS OF ACUPUNCTURE

Q: How reliably effective is acupuncture?

A: I think it is very reliable. It nearly always makes most people better to some degree. In a large percentage of people it gives a dramatic improvement, whatever their condition is.

Q: How will I feel after a treatment of acupuncture?

A: Most people feel relaxed and calm. Some people can feel a bit spaced out and disoriented. It is a good idea for them to go for a walk for a few minutes to ground themselves. It is certainly recommended not to rush straight back to work afterwards but instead chill out and enjoy the feeling!

Q: Will I feel instant results?

A: That is possible, yes. Sometimes when I'm putting needles in patients, they will fall asleep before I've finished installing the needles. That's how quickly a person can relax. Most people feel good when they leave the surgery, energised and more alert. But in the initial stages of the treatment this effect might only last a few hours to a few days. Over subsequent treatments the effect builds up and when treated weekly people generally feel better and better over a period of 8–10 weeks.

Q: Is acupuncture relaxing?
A: Yes! Nearly everyone, by the time they finish a session of Transformational Acupuncture, feels very relaxed. A lot of people fall asleep during treatment and wake up feeling quite refreshed, like a power nap. Depending on the specific situation, on occasions acupuncture can stir up feelings of restlessness and agitation. In most instances this settles before the end of the treatment.

On occasions, particularly early in the course of being treated, that feeling may last until the end of the session. This can be off-putting for the patient. Hang in there, though. Usually, that only occurs on one occasion. The next session is usually much more relaxing.

Q: How will I feel over the next day or two?
A: In most cases people feel an improvement immediately or over the next few hours. But I caution that some people do feel worse after a treatment and their symptoms are heightened. This is particularly common in the early stages of a course of treatment. I realise this can be off-putting for some people because it can feel unpleasant, but it's not very common. And when they have their next treatment that same feeling may happen again, but it's usually nowhere near as intense and over two or three treatments it will disappear. It's usually as a result of a big shift in the body, and the body doesn't like change; it likes going on its merry way, even if it's not doing the patient any good. Most people who get that kind of reaction will accept it's a part of the process and it's a good sign that things are changing. The worst situation, I suppose, is when people report absolutely nothing. No change in feeling or symptoms, whatsoever, better or worse, treatment after treatment.

Q: Why do I feel euphoric after acupuncture?

A: Acupuncture has been demonstrated to stimulate the release of endorphins, which are the body's natural morphine substance. Beta-endorphin has an anti-nociceptive effect, i.e. it decreases the feeling of pain. Gamma-endorphin is thought by researchers to have an anti-psychotic effect.

This might seem like a gross scientific experiment, but this nicely demonstrates that this is not a placebo effect, but an actual biochemical effect. In Beijing in the 60s and 70s, Professor Han Jisheng gave acupuncture to laboratory rats and measured the time it took for them to flick their tail away when a heat source was put underneath its tail. He demonstrated that the acupuncture was having a pain-relieving effect. He then killed those rats and extracted contents from their brains, and then injected the contents into other rats, which then also demonstrated a delayed tail-flick phenomenon. These results indicated the biochemical that had been extracted from the acupunctured rats and given to the non-acupunctured rat was having a pain-relieving effect, and this was later demonstrated to be beta-endorphin.

So yes, it is a real phenomenon, and beta-endorphin is the body's own morphine. It has a natural euphoric effect.

Q: Why do some sessions feel more intense or painful than others?

A: I guess it's to do with what the acupuncture treatment is trying to achieve in that session, which part of the body has the energy block. There are various points that have effects on the body and some points naturally seem to have a stronger effect than other points.

So, it all depends on the needles, the placement of the needles, and where the person is physically and mentally at the time. Treatments aren't always intense or painful. A particular point can be painful, or very uncomfortable, in one session. However, I could needle the exact same point in the next session a week later and the person could feel absolutely nothing. I think it's just that the intensity demonstrates that at that point the acupuncture needle is working hard to achieve homeostasis, or balance.

Q: Why do I sometimes feel restless during acupuncture, and sometimes feel calm and sleepy?

A: That is a good question. In my experience, when a person feels restless, it usually indicates there is liver involvement. The Chinese associate different emotions with different organs. The emotions associated with liver problems are anger, frustration, restlessness and irritability. This doesn't make sense from a Western medical viewpoint, but it does from the Chinese medical viewpoint. When one stimulates heart points, the person will often feel very calm, sleepy and even joyful.

Traditional Chinese medicine also likens the function of organs in the body to the various functions of government. It sees the heart as the emperor and the liver as the general of the army. The emperor, the heart, rules the body with benevolent love and has the interest of the whole body, the whole population, at heart and tries to do its best. When the general, the liver, listens to the emperor and carries out the emperor's plans, all is well in the body. The liver can get on with action and make things happen. When the liver, the general, is not listening to the heart, the emperor, the general's plans go astray. It loses battles, it doesn't have a clear strategy to win a war and then it gets angry and frustrated, and carries on quite a trip – and the person knows it because they feel angry, frustrated, irritable and restless.

This restless feeling that happens during a treatment can make the treatment feel like it goes on forever, but that doesn't happen too often. Most of the time, by the end of the treatment, that restlessness is gone and has been replaced by a calm peacefulness.

If the problem with the liver is deep-seated, it can take a number of treatments for that to ease. But when that shift happens, the person feels so much better and there's usually quite a shift in their mood through the following week.

PRACTITIONERS

Q: Is acupuncture performed by medical professionals?
A: Yes. Around 700 medical doctors perform acupuncture in Australia, as well as 2,000 non-medical acupuncturists.

If acupuncture is performed by a trained medical doctor, there is a Medicare rebate. Private health funds may cover other acupuncturists.

Q: How would I find a good practitioner?
A: There are two types of practitioners in Australia. First, there are those who are medical doctors who do acupuncture. Generally, these practitioners are members of the Australian Medical Acupuncture College, AMAC.

The remaining acupuncturists have trained at a university level in TCM, traditional Chinese medicine, and are generally members of the Acupuncture and Chinese Medicine Association of Australia, AACMA.

Both groups are highly trained. Their respective websites contain a list of practitioners by region.

For AMAC, visit:
www.amac.org.au/membership/?search&srchfield&paginate=1

For AACMA visit:
members.acupuncture.org.au/practitionersearch

Acupuncturists who have been trained in the method I've developed to treat mental health conditions, Transformational Acupuncture, can be found on our website: www.tai.healthcare

Q: Are acupuncturists registered, licensed and insured?
A: Yes, in Australia all acupuncturists (whether medical doctors or not) are registered with the Australian Health Practitioner Regulation Agency, AHPRA: www.ahpra.gov.au

One of the conditions of being registered is that they must have insurance. I caution to add that there are a number of people who are not registered, who don't necessarily claim to be acupuncturists, but they insert needles in people, so-called dry-needling, such as various massage therapists. This may help muscular problems, but it is not true acupuncture.

LENGTH OF TREATMENT

Q: How long is a session?
A: A Transformation Acupuncture session goes much longer than the traditional acupuncture treatment of 20 minutes. A session of Transformational Acupuncture lasts over an hour. Initially the person is treated with needles on the back of the body while they're lying face down. The needles are left to do their work for a period of 40 minutes. The needles are then removed and a second lot of needles are inserted on the front of the body while the patient lies face up for a further 20 minutes. It's a good idea to not have much on your agenda for the rest of that day. Just relax and enjoy the feeling.

Q: How many treatments will I need?
A: Generally, I would give a patient treatment once a week for about 10 weeks. As people improve and feel well for the full week,

I then look to treat them fortnightly. Often at this stage people will feel good for 8–10 days or so. Once they're feeling good for the whole fortnight I will treat them every three weeks, and so on. Regular patients get the ability to recognise when they need another treatment and book appointments accordingly.

Q: Will I need to keep coming for acupuncture indefinitely?

A: I have talked to patients many months or even a year or two after the treatment program has finished and they have remained well.

Q: Once I feel better, will I need maintenance treatments?

A: Sometimes yes, sometimes no. It depends what the person wants to achieve and how serious their problem is. The person will find out for themselves after a number of treatments how long the effect of treatment lasts. Several patients in my initial observational study, when followed up a year after having acupuncture, have not felt the need for further appointments.

Q: Why do some people with depression need ongoing maintenance treatments of acupuncture?

A: I think to a degree it depends on the type of depression the person has. Generally, depression falls into two groups: melancholic depression and non-melancholic depression. Melancholic depression is a chronic, pervasive depressed mood that often does not relate to anything that has happened in a person's life, not according to circumstances. This makes up only 10 per cent of patients with depression.

The clear majority, 90 per cent, have non-melancholic depression, which is often triggered in response to life's circumstances, such as a relationship breakup, a health crisis, a family crisis, and so forth, where they felt unable to cope. My impression is that these people no longer need maintenance treatment once they are feeling well again, off their antidepressants and are taught coping skills.

Whereas I think those who have a more pervasive, chronic depressed mood that has basically been life long would need ongoing maintenance treatments. Often post-traumatic stress disorder fits into this category.

OTHER COMMON QUESTIONS

Q: Is acupuncture beneficial for healthy people?
A: Even if a person feels well, they will feel even better after an acupuncture treatment! Stress and feeling uptight is such a common situation. Mood swings, irritability, and so forth, are helped by acupuncture.

Q: Can acupuncture help me lose weight?
A: That's a good question. I've never specifically quantified this. Being overweight or obese is a multifactorial condition of which the psyche is a part. I have had patients claim that they have lost weight because of the reduced need to comfort eat with reduction of feelings of depression and anxiety. But I wouldn't claim that as a direct effect of the acupuncture.

Q: Do I have to be a spiritual person for acupuncture to work?
A: Most definitely not. Acupuncture works no matter what your beliefs. One doesn't have to be a Buddhist or a Christian or believe in God for acupuncture to have its desired effect. One does not even have to believe in acupuncture for it to work! Like drug therapy, there is a placebo effect, but I've had many, many patients who have been quite skeptical of acupuncture and end up trying it because they felt they had run out of options. They are nearly always pleasantly surprised at how well acupuncture works and find they become converts.

Q: Can acupuncture change my views on life, or change the way I think or feel?

A: That's a good question. I believe it can. My first experience of receiving acupuncture was mind-blowing. I couldn't believe the profound shift in the way I felt in a matter of minutes from just having some very fine stainless-steel needles placed in various parts of my body. I would not have credited it as having that kind of effect, so powerful and immediate, without having experienced it myself. If a patient has clinical depression and has regular treatments and their depression leaves, I can't believe that it wouldn't change the way the person thinks and feels or change their views on life in general.

Q: Does what I eat affect how the acupuncture works?

A: I guess it's not a good idea to have an acupuncture treatment just having eaten a big, rich meal. But I think regardless of a person's diet, acupuncture will work. However, there are dietary strategies to help a person with depression and that includes what foods to eat and what foods to avoid.

CONCLUSION

One thing I have discovered about myself is that I would much rather read a book than write a book. I can easily set aside an hour or two to read a good book, but come up with every excuse why I can't find time to write another chapter. Every time, though, I feel compelled to write because of the stories I hear from my patients. Virtually every day my patients tell me how acupuncture has changed their lives.

For instance, I recently had a patient come in requesting acupuncture for pain relief. The pain was between her shoulder blades and aggravated by her work as a hairdresser. I noted on her file that she had been coming to our practice on and off for a few years, often for management of depression and had been referred on a number of occasions to several different psychologists and a mindfulness-based stress reduction program. After her acupuncture session she said that she felt totally present and had been aware of a number of unusual sensations on one side of her body only. She had also been thinking clearly and had decided to quit hairdressing and study trauma counselling! This revelation had come to her in her first acupuncture session. The next week I asked her had she had any further thoughts following her acupuncture session, and she said that she had already tendered her resignation with the hairdressing salon. That's what I call getting your life back naturally!

Tell me the name of a painkiller or a procedure that would be as effective as the kind of treatment that the acupuncture gave her. Painkillers merely kill the pain, but they don't correct the problem that causes the pain. Her pain was a message her body and subconscious mind were trying to tell her about her work as a hairdresser. And not even about her physical work as such, but a deeper message that her work as a hairdresser – although giving her an income and occupying her time for many hours a week – was not fulfilling her mission in life.

In fact, a painkiller would have numbed the message her body and subconscious mind was sending her and postpone the day that she took action to remove the real cause of her pain. Transformational Acupuncture, on the other hand, helped her to focus mind, body and spirit to be as one, and see the connection between the pain resulting from the chronic tension between her shoulders with her underlying dissatisfaction with her hairdressing work and not getting on with her greater mission in life as a trauma counsellor.

As I said, I hear these sorts of stories all the time from my patients receiving Transformational Acupuncture. I recently surveyed seventy of my patients about their experience of Transformational Acupuncture over a period of eight weeks. Of those who responded to open-ended questions, 93% reported that acupuncture had affected them in a positive way. 49% reported feeling more relaxed and 40% said that they had a spiritual experience or an emotional release. 37% experienced relief of physical or mental discomfort. No one reported any adverse effects. Those seem like good odds to me. Maybe you would benefit, too?

Discover more about how Transformational Acupuncture can change your life today at https://stickittodepression.com

ABOUT ALEXANDER JOANNOU

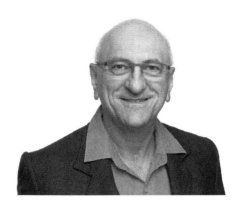

Dr Alexander Joannou MBBS(Hons) FACNEM is creator of the Transformational Acupuncture System and founder of Northside Health a ten-doctor medical centre.

He is a conjoint lecturer with UNSW and an RACGP-accredited supervisor and has been training medical students, international medical graduates and General Practice Registrars for 20 years.

He has learned a lot about the human psyche in his 40-year medical career. With around 300,000 patient consultations, including performing over 50,000 acupuncture treatments, Dr Alex has witnessed firsthand the complex interrelationship between mind, body and spirit.

In conjunction with the Southern Cross University, he is researching the benefits of acupuncture on a range of mental illnesses. With over one million Australians living with depression he is on a mission to train acupuncturists and to raise awareness with medical doctors, to make a difference in the world.

He is author of the companion book, *Stick it to Depression: Another Tool in Your Doctor's Bag* to make medical doctors aware of the benefits of acupuncture in managing depression and anxiety. You can reach him at DrAlex@TAI.Healthcare or at linkedin.com/in/dralexjoannou/

ACKNOWLEDGEMENTS

I thank God and acknowledge the following people for continuing to support me on this journey.

The 'Word Witch', Dixie Carlton, who helped me unpack what was in my head, and who has coached, cajoled and encouraged me throughout the process of writing this book.

Ann Wilson, and all at Indie Experts, for transforming my notes into a book.

My patients, especially those whose stories are in this book, who have me taught me much about the human spirit in the face of all kinds of adversity. Many have been just as enthusiastic about acupuncture as me.

Andrew Griffith, author extraordinaire, who made me see that it was possible to write a book and gave me the concrete steps to do it.

Dr Mikio Sankey, who speaks few words, but each is a gem. Every conversation I have with him is inspiring. He opened my mind to see the possibilities of acupuncture for mental health.

Alison Clarke-Daly, for showing me that acupuncture points are palpably real.

My Ruby Rose, who inspired me to take what I was discovering seriously and to document it.

OTHER BOOKS BY ALEXANDER JOANNOU

STICK IT TO DEPRESSION: ANOTHER TOOL IN YOUR DOCTOR'S BAG

WHO has now ranked depression as the number one cause of ill-health and disability in the world, and estimate it's affecting more than 300 million people in the world. That's only counting those who actually suffer from it – it does not include the many hundreds of millions more families, co-workers, and friends who are also in their way living with the effects of depression in their own lives too. The impact of this condition is incalculable.

Running a medical practice featuring the Transformational Acupuncture System keeps Dr Alexander Joannou very busy. Helping to spread the word about the benefits of using acupuncture as a trusted tool in any GP's medical bag is a passion that has grown out of his own experiences of success using this option – not only for himself, but with his patients too.

This companion book to *Stick It to Depression: Get Your Life Back, Naturally* challenges modern GPs to consider and implement ancient Eastern medicine in the form of acupuncture in the management of depression and anxiety.

These two books are designed to help patients and doctors

engage in meaningful conversation about considering using acupuncture as an adjunct in the treatment of depression.

If you or someone you care about is struggling to live with depression, find out more about what this really means, why so many people are in this predicament and what we can do to bring about real change rather than put a band aid on the symptoms.

Please follow Dr Alex on Facebook, Linkedin and his website www.TAI.Healthcare

ENDNOTES

1 https://apps.who.int/iris/handle/10665/41864
2 https://www.ausstats.abs.gov.au/ausstats/subscriber.
   nsf/0/6AE6DA447F985FC2CA2574EA00122BD6/$File/National%20
   Survey%20of%20Mental%20Health%20and%20Wellbeing%20Summary%20
   of%20Results.pdf
3 https://www.who.int/news-room/detail/09-09-2019-suicide-one-person-dies-
   every-40-seconds
4 https://www.who.int/mental_health/in_the_workplace/en/
5 https://www.weforum.org/agenda/2015/02/the-link-between-unemployment-
   and-suicide
6 https://www.weforum.org/agenda/2019/06/bad-economic-news-increases-
   suicide-rates-new-research/
7 https://www.beyondblue.org.au/who-does-it-affect/men/what-causes-anxiety-
   and-depression-in-men/alcohol-and-drug-use
8 https://www.researchgate.net/publication/50303291_Alcohol_and_depression
9 https://www.racgp.org.au/afp/2012/may/smoking-and-depression/
10 https://journals.lww.com/neuroreport/Abstract/2002/07020/Effect_of_
   nicotine_and_nicotinic_receptors_on.6.aspx
11 https://www.ncbi.nlm.nih.gov/pmc/articles/PMC2902727/
12 http://www.annfammed.org/content/14/1/54.full
13 Ibid.
14 https://www.diabetesaustralia.com.au/depression-and-mental-health
15 https://www.jdrf.org/t1d-resources/living-with-t1d/mental-health/
   depression/#:~:text=Depression%20is%20estimated%20to%20affect,who%20
   do%20not%20have%20T1D.
16 https://jamanetwork.com/journals/jamainternalmedicine/fullarticle/207998

17 https://www.ncbi.nlm.nih.gov/pubmed/26921864
18 https://www.ncbi.nlm.nih.gov/pubmed/23724696
19 http://apsychoserver.psych.arizona.edu/JJBAReprints/PSYC621/Blashfield_
    etal_2014_ARCP.pdf
20 https://www.beyondblue.org.au/the-facts/anxiety/types-of-anxiety/social-phobia
21 https://www.psychology.org.au/publications/inpsych/2012/february/
    manicavasagar
22 https://www.blackdoginstitute.org.au/news/news-detail/2017/08/21/what-
    causes-depression-what-we-know-don-t-know-and-suspect
23 https://www.ncbi.nlm.nih.gov/pmc/articles/PMC3955126/
24 https://www.cdc.gov/ncbddd/adhd/timeline.html
25 https://www.aph.gov.au/About_Parliament/Parliamentary_Departments/
    Parliamentary_Library/FlagPost/2011/January/Large_increase_in_stimulant_
    use_for_ADHD_in_Australia_new_study
26 https://www.mja.com.au/journal/2017/206/2/influence-birth-month-
    probability-western-australian-children-being-treated-adhd
27 http://www.health.wa.gov.au/publications/documents/MICADHD_Raine_
    ADHD_Study_report_022010.pdf
28 https://adaa.org/understanding-anxiety/related-illnesses/other-related-
    conditions/adult-adhd
29 https://www.apa.org/monitor/2012/06/prescribing.aspx
30 https://www.ncbi.nlm.nih.gov/pmc/articles/PMC4172306/
31 https://www.frontiersin.org/articles/10.3389/fpsyt.2020.00478/full
32 ibid.
33 https://www.statnews.com/2016/06/08/antidepressants-teens-kids/
34 https://www.aihw.gov.au/getmedia/d35a03a3-1500-4775-b3e1-9a99f3168bb8/
    Mental-health-related-prescriptions-2016-17.pdf.aspx
35 https://www.ncbi.nlm.nih.gov/pmc/articles/PMC4970636/
36 https://www.ausdoc.com.au/news/incredibly-unhelpful-antidepressant-guide-
    lines-need-urgent-update-0
37 https://thenewdaily.com.au/life/auto/2018/07/30/takata-airbag-recall-website/
38 https://www.medscape.com/medline/abstract/16428706
39 https://www.ncbi.nlm.nih.gov/pubmed/8092546
40 https://www.newscientist.com/article/dn6918-up-to-140000-heart-attacks-
    linked-to-vioxx/
41 https://www.ncbi.nlm.nih.gov/pubmed/11686961
42 http://apps.who.int/medicinedocs/en/d/Js22276en/
43 https://www.thennt.com/nnt/statins-persons-low-risk-cardiovascular-disease/
44 https://www.ncbi.nlm.nih.gov/pubmed/6100743
45 https://www.ncbi.nlm.nih.gov/pmc/articles/PMC3987289/
46 https://jeb.biologists.org/content/jexbio/213/18/3081.full.pdf

47 https://www.ncbi.nlm.nih.gov/pubmed/10829090

48 https://www.intechopen.com/books/serotonin-a-chemical-messenger-between-all-types-of-living-cells/production-and-function-of-serotonin-in-cardiac-cells

49 https://www.heartmath.org/research/science-of-the-heart/energetic-communication/ https://www.heartmath.org/research/science-of-the-heart/energetic-communication/

50 https://pubmed.ncbi.nlm.nih.gov/20034389/ Is Psychiatry the least popular specialty for UK and international medical graduates?

51 https://digital.nhs.uk/data-and-information/publications/statistical/quality-and-outcomes-framework-achievement-prevalence-and-exceptions-data/2018-19-pas

52 https://www.thelancet.com/journals/lancet/article/PIIS0140-6736(17)32802-7/fulltext#seccestitle140

53 https://www.thelancet.com/journals/lanpsy/article/PIIS2215-0366(19)30215-9/fulltext

54 https://bmcmedicine.biomedcentral.com/articles/10.1186/s12916-017-0791-y

55 https://journals.plos.org/plosone/article?id=10.1371/journal.pone.0222768

56 https://link.springer.com/chapter/10.1007%2F978-3-642-10857-0_5

57 https://yosan.edu/wp-content/uploads/2018/05/A-Guide-to-Regulating-Hormone-Function-Utilizing-Traditional-Chinese-Medicine-by-Nefertiti-Abdou.pdf

58 https://www.ncbi.nlm.nih.gov/pmc/articles/PMC6276442/

59 https://academic.oup.com/qjmed/article/107/5/341/1563714

60 https://doi.org/10.1136/bmj.h2435

61 https://doi.org/10.1016/S0254-6272(15)30132-1

Made in the USA
Middletown, DE
09 December 2022

17835515R00091